SUPERFOODS
HAPPINESS

First published in French in 2015 by Les Publications Modus Vivendi Inc.
under the title *Superaliments bonheur*.
© Elisabeth Cerqueira, Marise Charron and Les Publications Modus Vivendi Inc., 2017

MODUS VIVENDI PUBLISHING INC.

55 Jean-Talon Street West
Montreal, Quebec H2R 2W8
CANADA

modusvivendipublishing.com

Publisher: Marc G. Alain
Editorial director: Isabelle Jodoin
Content and copy editor: Nolwenn Gouezel
English-language editor: Carol Sherman
Translator: Rhonda Mullins
English-language copy editor: Maeve Haldane
Graphic designer: Émilie Houle
Food photographer: André Noël (anoelphoto.com)
Food stylist: Gabrielle Dalessandro
Authors' and superfoods photographer: Camille Gyrya (www.camillegyrya.com)

Additional photography:
Pages 5, 19 and 41: Dreamstime.com
Pages 8, 10, 17, 22, 31, 56, 57, 58, 59, 61, 62, 65, 66, 194, 208 and 214: iStock

ISBN: 978-1-77286-034-4 (PAPERBACK)

ISBN: 978-1-77286-035-1 (PDF)
ISBN: 978-1-77286-036-8 (EPUB)
ISBN: 978-1-77286-037-5 (KINDLE)

Legal deposit – Bibliothèque et Archives nationales du Québec, 2017
Legal deposit – Library and Archives Canada, 2017

Government of Quebec – Tax Credit for Book Publishing – Program administered by SODEC

Funded by the Government of Canada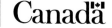

Printed in Canada

SUPERFOODS
HAPPINESS

Over 50 recipes to improve your mood and start smiling

ELISABETH CERQUEIRA AND MARISE CHARRON, RD

With the collaboration of Nolwenn Gouezel

MODUS VIVENDI

CONTENTS

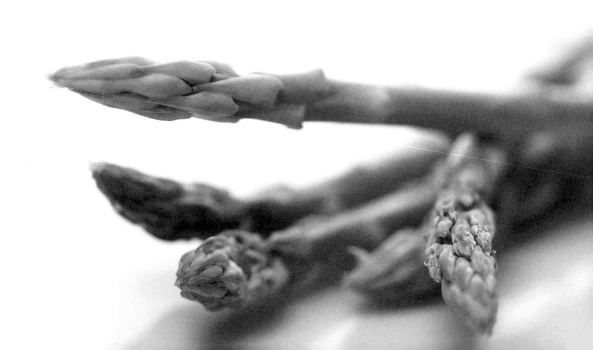

THE AUTHORS

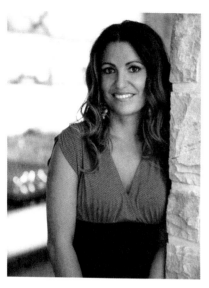

ELISABETH CERQUEIRA

Elisabeth Cerqueira is co-president of NutriSimple, a network of over 50 private nutrition clinics in Quebec. She is the coauthor of the **Superfoods** series and two books in the **Know What To Eat** series: *Weight Loss* and *Arthritis* and *Inflammation*. She has a bachelor's degree in nutrition from McGill University and is a member of the Ordre professionnel des diététistes du Québec (Professional College of Dietitians of Quebec).

For over 15 years, Elisabeth has been teaching clients to eat by helping them increase the nutritional value of their food. She treats nutritional imbalances that lead to obesity, diabetes, cholesterol, arthritis, anorexia and more. Her mission is to be her clients' partner in health. At the leading edge of scientific research, she and her team of dietitians offer a simple nutritional program. Her empirical approach promotes a diet that helps clients get in peak shape. She is known for her passion for nutrition in medical circles and in the arts. She is a dietitian to a number of celebrities, including Gerard Butler in the movie *300*.

Elisabeth loves to cook with her three children and applies the principles in this book on a daily basis. She believes that eating well should be a simple pleasure. From a European background, she fully enjoys all that life has to offer, including food.

elisabeth@nutrisimple.com
nutrisimple.com

6

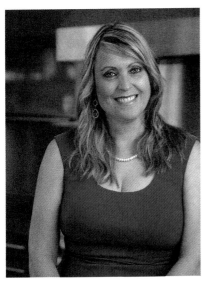

MARISE CHARRON

Marise Charron graduated in nutrition from Laval University and has been a practicing dietitian for over 20 years. She is the author of a number of successful cookbooks and loves to share her knowledge of nutrition and cooking, two related areas that she is passionate about. Marise loves discovering and inventing new recipes and believes that eating well means savoring the moment.

In 1991, Marise founded the Groupe Harmonie Santé to provide professional development to dietitians in private practice and promote discussion among health care professionals. In 2010, she teamed up with Elisabeth Cerqueira to create NutriSimple.

An entrepreneur at heart, she is also at the helm of Nutrition2C (nutrition2c.com), which offers a nutritional analysis and labeling service to companies, schools, restaurants and magazines. In 1998, the Ordre professionnel des diététistes du Québec (Professional College of Dietitians of Quebec) recognized her work with the Annual Merit Award in Nutrition.

As a clinical dietitian, Marise loves the close relationships she develops with her clients, recommending healthy habits using an approach that respects body diversity.

marise@nutrisimple.com
nutrisimple.com

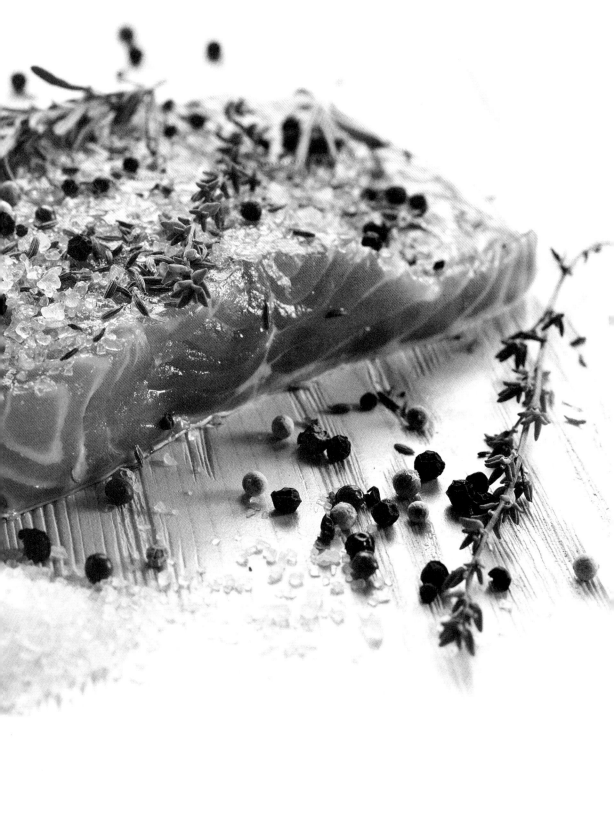

INTRODUCTION

Mood swings, low morale and irritability are problems that should not be taken lightly. They end up making people more vulnerable and sensitive to stress, and they can lead to depression, a serious pathological condition that affects 121 million people worldwide.

According to many studies, mood can be influenced by lifestyle, particularly diet. A diet that includes a wide variety of unprocessed foods (vegetables, fruit, fish, nuts, legumes) and that includes good fats, such as those found in the Mediterranean diet, could reduce the symptoms of depression. And a diet with too much processed food has a negative effect on mood.

This book explains how to keep smiling through a customized diet. Twenty superfoods have been selected for their nutritional value. By definition, superfoods are foods that have more nutrients and health benefits than other foods. As part of a varied, balanced diet, they offer particular nutritional benefits.

The superfoods presented in this book are good sources of nutrients with scientifically proven properties to help improve your mood. Read through the glossary to find out more about these happiness allies. As part of a healthy, balanced diet, these superfoods can promote well-being and calm, stabilize mood, reduce irritability, fight chronic stress, restore energy and relieve symptoms of depression.

Learn how to choose, store and prepare food to get the most nutrients out of it and get the most out of your diet. And discover more than 50 healthy recipes that contain one or more of the top 20 happiness superfoods.

See your doctor if your symptoms of depression persist.

NOTE

No one food alone contains all the nutrients a body needs. This is why a healthy, balanced diet is essential for good health. Don't limit your diet to a few superfoods — no matter what their concentration of nutrients — even if they have vitamins and minerals with scientifically proven properties. Include them in your diet, but aim for variety and balance.

THE CHEMISTRY OF HAPPINESS:
THE ESSENTIAL ROLE OF DIET

The feeling of happiness is closely related to neurotransmitters, chemical messages that ensure the proper functioning of the brain. Without neurotransmitters, we would have no memory or emotions. The two main neurotransmitters for well-being are serotonin and dopamine. Research has shown that diet can have a direct influence on mood, naturally stimulating the secretion of neurotransmitters.

Proteins, made up of amino acids, are the essential building blocks for these neurotransmitters. Vitamins also come into their creation (including B_{12} and folate), as do trace elements (including magnesium and selenium). Consuming these nutrients could increase the amount of neurotransmitters available to the brain. If you don't get enough nutrients, there are fewer secretions and morale drops. That said, the influence of diet on mood comes from the synergy of a number of nutrients from different food sources rather than from a specific, isolated nutrient.

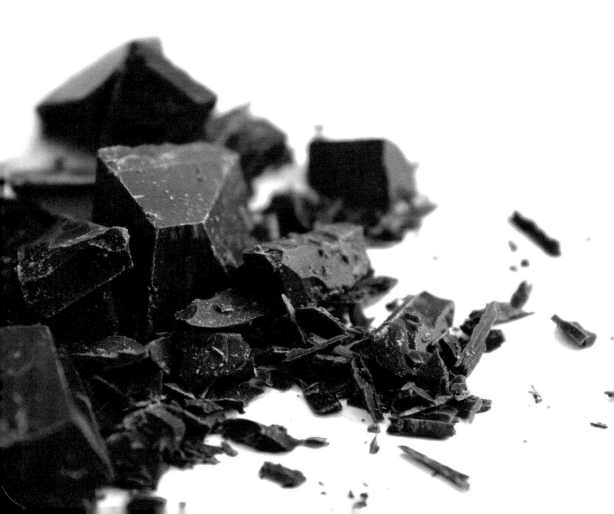

SEROTONIN

Serotonin, sometimes called the "happiness hormone," plays an essential role in creating a sense of well-being. It promotes relaxation, a good mood, serenity, appetite and sleep, while reducing tension, aggressiveness and anger. High serotonin levels can induce calm, careful and considered behavior. Abnormally low levels may be associated with irritability, impulsiveness and aggressiveness.

Certain foods contain precious amino acids and vitamins that stimulate the secretion of serotonin. For example, eating foods rich in tryptophan (an amino acid) can increase serotonin levels in the body. But for this to happen, the body needs vitamins (mainly those from the B group, such as B_6) and carbohydrates. (The best sources of these nutrients are included in the *10 Tips for a Good Mood*, p. 12.) Afternoon snack and evening mealtime are periods conducive to the secretion of serotonin.

DOPAMINE

Dopamine, sometimes called the "pleasure hormone," is the neurotransmitter responsible for keeping the brain alert and active. It is also involved in mood stabilization. High dopamine levels promote adventurous behavior, a quest for pleasure and strong emotions, as well as sexual pleasure. Abnormally low levels may be associated with a lack of motivation, melancholy and feeling emotionally flat.

The availability of dopamine in the body depends essentially on your intake of tyrosine and phenylalanine, two amino acids that are found in dark chocolate, bananas, avocados, almonds, pumpkin seeds, lentils and other protein-based foods. Eating food rich in tyrosine and phenylalanine promotes the secretion of dopamine in the body, provided there are sufficient levels of vitamins (mainly those from the B group, including B_6, contained, for example, in salmon, sweet potatoes, spinach and bananas). Breakfast and lunch are periods conducive to the secretion of dopamine.

10 TIPS
FOR A GOOD MOOD

1
CONSUME OMEGA-3S THREE TIMES A WEEK

Choose omega-3s from marine rather than plant sources. According to scientific studies, cultures that regularly consume fatty fish (such as tuna, salmon, mackerel, sardines, herring and trout) have less risk of severe depression than those that consume little or none. Omega-3s from plant sources, such as walnuts, should not be neglected, even though they have less of an effect on mood.

2
INCREASE YOUR CONSUMPTION OF TRYPTOPHAN

Your brain transforms tryptophan (an amino acid) into serotonin. This neurotransmitter plays an important role in regulating sleep, appetite and mood (see *The Chemistry of Happiness*, p. 10). It is found abundantly in foods such as poultry, fish, dairy products, nuts, peanuts and bananas.

3
COUNT ON B COMPLEX VITAMINS

High consumption of dietary sources of tryptophan combined with vitamin B_6 (found, for example, in bananas, sweet potatoes, avocados, salmon, sunflower seeds and legumes) can promote the synthesis of serotonin, thereby reducing the symptoms of depression. The best sources are spinach, asparagus, avocados, beets and legumes. Blood levels low in vitamin B_{12} may be associated with an increased risk of depression. Sardines, salmon and eggs are excellent sources.

4
CHOOSE UNREFINED CARBOHYDRATES

To function, our brains have a constant need for carbohydrates, because they do not store any reserves. Choose whole-grain products. Also choose carbohydrates from vegetables (such as sweet potato), fruits, legumes, milk and substitutes. The evening meal should ideally provide the body with more carbohydrates than animal proteins.

5
MAINTAIN A HIGH INTAKE OF VITAMIN D

More and more studies suggest a correlation between depression and the level of vitamin D in the blood. Vitamin D could, in fact, increase the production of serotonin. Since the sun is the main source of vitamin D, it is hard to get when you live at a latitude that does not enable the body to produce any between October and March. So it is a good idea to regularly consume food high in vitamin D: fatty fish, egg yolk and food enriched with vitamin D.

6 LOOK FOR IRON, MAGNESIUM AND SELENIUM

These three minerals play a role in alleviating symptoms of depression. For instance, iron and magnesium deficiencies could aggravate the fatigue associated with depression. According to a number of studies, those with a selenium deficiency run a greater risk of suffering from mood disorders than others.

7 DRINK GREEN TEA AND COFFEE, BUT NOT TOO MUCH

Rich in polyphenols, green tea helps maintain a stable mood. However, too much tea can reduce the absorption of iron. So it's best to drink it between meals. As for coffee, a study conducted of 50,000 middle-aged women established that the risk of developing depression was reduced by 20% in those who drank four cups of coffee per day compared with those who drank less. But take note: beyond this amount, caffeine can cause anxiety.

8 DON'T SKIP MEALS AND STAY HYDRATED

Not skipping meals stabilizes sugar levels in the blood. Blood sugar levels that rise and fall can result in irritability and mood swings. According to a number of studies, a nutritious breakfast that includes protein-rich food (such as eggs, cheese or Greek yogurt) and food rich in fiber (such as whole-grain cereal and fruit) helps improve mood. Plus drinking about 1 to 2 liters (4 to 8 cups) of fluids per day prevents dehydration that can result in fatigue, an inability to concentrate and even dizziness.

9 GET ENOUGH SLEEP

It has been shown that there is a correlation between sleep disturbances and depression. Sleep seven to eight hours and try to go to bed and get up at regular hours, even on the weekend.

10 GET MOVING EVERY DAY

According to many studies conducted among people diagnosed with depression, regular physical activity may have a similar effect as taking an antidepressant. Although the underlying mechanism is still unknown, we do know that exercising regularly (for 20 minutes three or four times a week) stabilizes mood, increases energy and helps reduce stress.

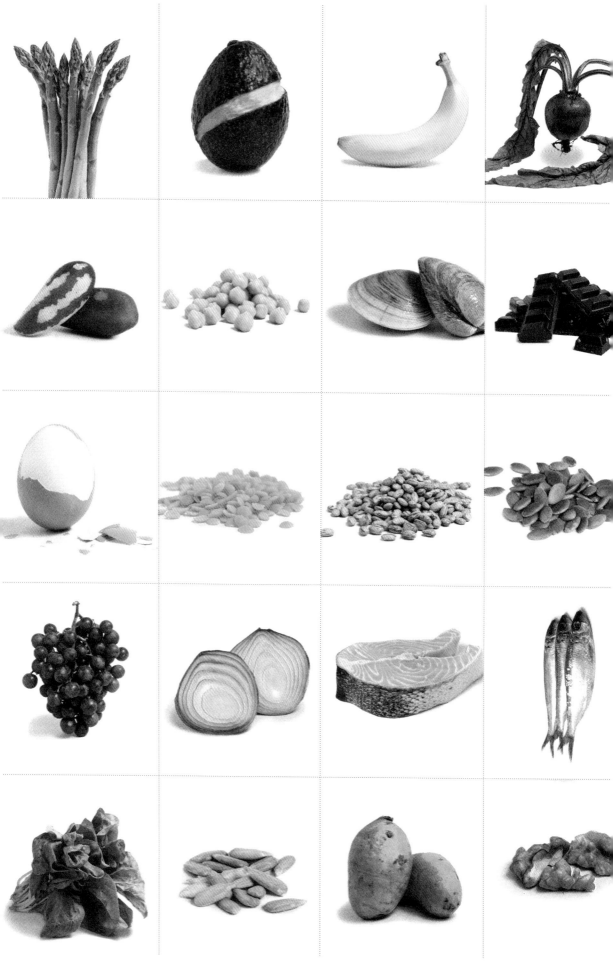

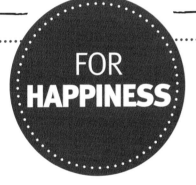

20 SUPERFOODS

FOR HAPPINESS

ASPARAGUS

Composition

EXCELLENT SOURCE OF: vitamin K, folate

GOOD SOURCE OF: iron

SOURCE OF: fiber, vitamins A, B_1, B_2, B_3, B_6, C and vitamin E (when boiled), copper, manganese, potassium, selenium (when boiled)

Asparagus contains tryptophan.

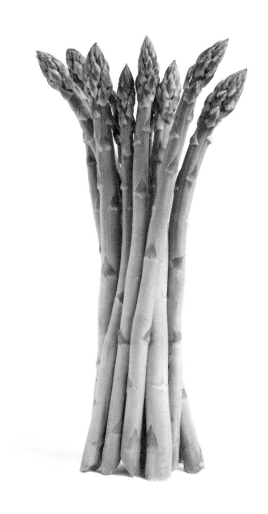

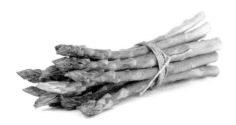

In ancient times, asparagus was attributed with many medicinal properties. It was used to cure all sorts of illnesses, from rheumatism to toothaches. These days it is thought to be a purifying agent, a diuretic and sometimes even an aphrodisiac.

VIRTUES

Improving mood

Asparagus ranks fifth among foods for folate content. Studies suggest a correlation between eating plenty of food rich in folate and a reduced risk of depression. According to the findings from a Harvard University study, 38% of women with depression have a folate deficiency. Plus, folate may reinforce the effect of antidepressants.

Encouraging well-being

Eating asparagus may have a positive influence on mood, appetite and sleep, because it is a source not only of tryptophan (an amino acid), but also of vitamins, which together promote the secretion of serotonin (see *The Chemistry of Happiness*, p. 10).

THINGS TO REMEMBER

- Five cooked asparagus meet about 25% of daily folate needs for the general population.

- Cooking, canning or freezing vegetables reduces their folate content.

- The vitamins and minerals are particularly concentrated in the tips of asparagus.

- Green asparagus are richer in vitamins and minerals than white ones, which grow underground, never seeing the sun. This is why they do not turn green.

BUYING AND STORING

- The stalk must be firm, easy to snap and dry at the end, and the tip must be a nice color, tightly closed and compact. Do not choose asparagus with grayish ends.

- Raw asparagus doesn't keep well: keep it in bundles, wrapped in a damp paper towel in a plastic bag. Place it in the vegetable crisper in the refrigerator. To make the most of its nutrients, eat it soon after buying, because it quickly becomes woody.

HOW TO EAT IT

Raw: cut in thin strips and served with vinaigrette.

Cooked: boiled, steamed (served hot or cold with a vinaigrette or sauce), roasted in the oven (served with olive oil, garlic and lemon), in soup, risottos, frittatas, sautés, quiches or vegetable muffins.

AVOCADO

Composition

EXCELLENT SOURCE OF: vitamin K, folate, fiber
GOOD SOURCE OF: vitamins B_5, B_6, C and E
SOURCE OF: copper, magnesium, potassium

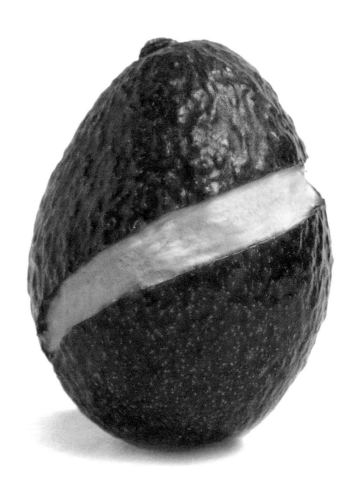

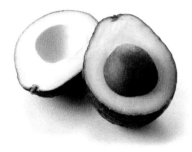

While avocado is often considered a vegetable, it is actually a fruit, specifically the reproductive organ of the avocado tree. Its name is derived from the Aztec word ahuacalt, which means "testicle," referring to the shape of the fruit and the fact that it hangs in pairs.

VIRTUES

Regulating mood

Avocados are an excellent source of folate, a vitamin that is essential to the proper functioning of the nervous system. A sufficient intake in folate regulates mood and reduces the risk of irritability.

Fighting depression

Avocado is a good source of vitamins B_5 and B_6, which help transform tryptophan into serotonin. The vitamins and the amino acid work together to regulate mood and therefore may help fight depression.

Increasing energy

Having energy helps get in a good mood. A source of fat and protein, avocado is a high-energy food; it is one of the fruits that is highest in protein (2 g per 100 g serving, ½ avocado).

THINGS TO REMEMBER

• The Hass variety is the richest in folate.

• A half an avocado meets 24% of the daily needs in fiber and 30% of daily needs in vitamin C.

• Unlike other sources of fat, avocado contains soluble fiber, which is an effective ally in stabilizing blood sugar, and insoluble fiber, which promotes intestinal transit and makes you feel satisfied.

HOW TO EAT IT

• In guacamole, mousse, smoothies, salads and sandwiches.

• Stuffed with seafood or chicken.

────── CHEF'S TIPS ──────

• Wrap avocado in newspaper if you want it to ripen faster.

• Roll avocado in your hands for a few minutes to make it easier to peel.

• As soon as it is peeled, sprinkle with lemon or lime juice to stop it from turning black, because it is sensitive to oxidation.

BANANA

Composition

GOOD SOURCE OF: vitamin B_6, manganese

SOURCE OF: vitamins B_2, B_5 and C, folate, magnesium, potassium, copper, fiber

Banana contains tryptophan and dopamine.

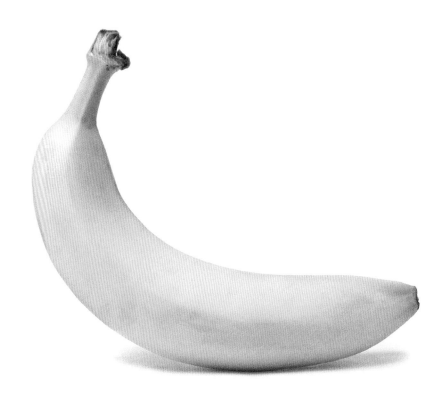

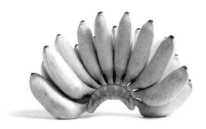

In India, bananas are nicknamed "fruit of paradise," because, according to legend, Eve offered Adam a banana and not an apple. Regardless, it is not a forbidden fruit. Because of its shape, the banana is a symbol of good humor.

VIRTUES

Stabilizing mood
Bananas are a good source of vitamin B_6, which is essential to the secretion of serotonin. Eating them helps regulate mood, sleep and appetite.

Relieving symptoms of depression during menopause
Studies show that bananas can relieve the symptoms of depression that some women suffer from during menopause.

THINGS TO REMEMBER

• The Cavendish variety, by far the most popular, contains dopamine, sometimes called the "pleasure hormone" (see *The Chemistry of Happiness*, p. 10).

• The riper the banana, the sweeter the taste, because the starch turns into sugar as the banana ripens. A ripe banana may contain the equivalent of 5 tsp of sugar, and it is much easier to digest than a green banana.

BUYING, STORING AND PREPARING

• A banana is ripe when it is still firm, bright yellow, even at the ends, with no brown marks.

• Bananas are stored at room temperature. To ripen faster, wrap them in a paper bag and leave them at room temperature. Cold slows the ripening and blackens the peel.

• Peel overripe bananas and keep them in the freezer.

• Bananas blacken quickly once peeled. Sprinkle them with lemon juice to prevent oxidation.

HOW TO EAT IT

Raw: in brochettes, fruit salad, tapioca, cold cereal or oat bran, frozen with a dark chocolate coating with ginger and crushed walnuts, in sorbet or puréed.

Cooked: flambéed, sautéed, in muffins, pancakes, cake or bread.

```
──────── DRIED BANANA ────────

Dried banana has three times more sugar, minerals and trace elements than
the fresh variety. Vitamins and minerals are four to five times more concentrated,
except vitamin C, which is destroyed in dehydration.
```

BEETS

Composition

EXCELLENT SOURCE OF: folate

GOOD SOURCE OF: manganese

SOURCE OF: fiber, vitamins B$_3$ and C, potassium, magnesium, iron

Beets contain uridine, betaine and tryptophan.

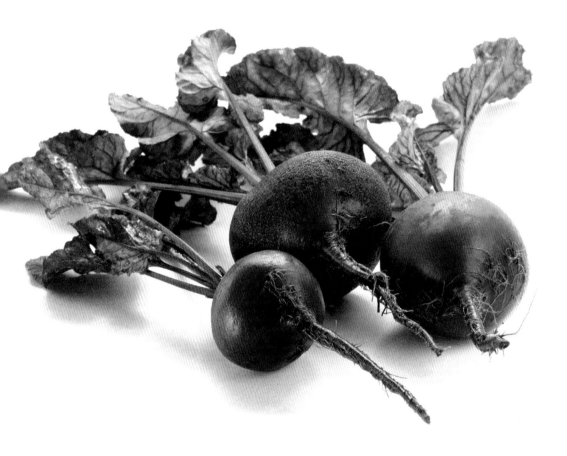

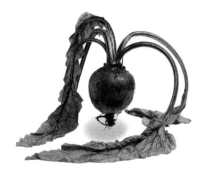

Beets are root vegetables, like carrots and turnips. Today we mainly eat the beetroot, but it used to be that only the stems were eaten. The root was used exclusively as a remedy for headaches and toothaches.

VIRTUES

Encouraging a good mood
Raw red beets are an excellent source of folate. Studies suggest a correlation between eating plenty of foods rich in folate and a reduced risk of depression, particularly in men.

Having potentially antidepressant effects
Beets contain betaine and uridine, substances that have potentially antidepressive effects and that promote the natural secretion of dopamine and serotonin by the body.

Improving mood
Beets are a good source of tryptophan, an amino acid the body transforms into serotonin. This neurotransmitter regulates sleep, appetite and mood.

THINGS TO REMEMBER

• Beets are one of the vegetables highest in sugar.

• To preserve the folate, which is sensitive to heat, beets should be cooked unpeeled or eaten raw.

STORING
Beets should be stored in the refrigerator in a perforated plastic bag.

HOW TO EAT IT
Raw: grated in salads (they go nicely with apples, oranges, goat cheese and nuts), in juice or in smoothies.

Cooked: roasted, boiled, marinated in vinegar, cooked on the barbecue en papillote, in soup (borscht), as a side for game or red meat or as chips.

CHEF'S TIPS

• Beet greens can be cooked with a bit of oil or eaten in a salad like spinach or Swiss chard.

• After peeling beets, clean your hands with lemon juice to get rid of stains.

BRAZIL NUTS

Composition

EXCELLENT SOURCE OF: selenium, magnesium, copper, phosphorus

GOOD SOURCE OF: vitamins B_1 and E, manganese, zinc

SOURCE OF: iron, potassium, calcium, fiber, protein

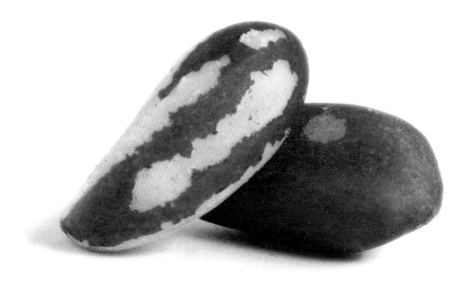

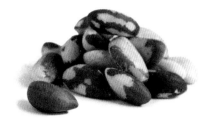

This fruit of the Brazil nut tree originally comes from the Amazon. Despite their name, the most significant exporter of Brazil nuts is Bolivia, where they are called *nuez de Brasil*. And though it is commonly called the Brazil nut, in botanical terms it is the seed from the fruit of this tree.

VIRTUES

Reducing the risk of depression

The Brazil nut definitely leads the pack of foods high in selenium. A deficiency in food-derived selenium can be associated with irritability and anxiety and increases the risk of depression. Eating two Brazil nuts daily increases selenium in the blood by 65%.

Fighting the effects of stress

Regularly eating food rich in magnesium (like the Brazil nut) promotes relaxation and restorative sleep, particularly since it helps fight anxiety and agitation by countering the secretion of cortisol, the hormone released in times of stress.

THINGS TO REMEMBER

- Brazil nuts are very satisfying.

- Most of the fat in Brazil nuts is good fat: almost 70% is polyunsaturated fat.

- The Brazil nut is a complete source of protein, because it has all the amino acids essential to tissue growth and repair.

- You can easily use Brazil nuts instead of coconut in recipes.

BUYING AND STORING

It is a good idea to buy Brazil nuts in the shell or at least with the brown skin on. They keep in their shell for about two months in a dark, dry place. If shelled, they keep in a sealed container for two to four weeks at room temperature or for nine months in the refrigerator.

HOW TO EAT IT

- Plain as a snack (in trail mix with dried fruit), in a green or mixed salad.

- With rice or couscous, in stuffing and sautés.

CHICKPEAS

Composition

EXCELLENT SOURCE OF: folate, manganese, copper, iron, fiber, protein

GOOD SOURCE OF: phosphorus

SOURCE OF: vitamins B_1 and B_6, zinc, magnesium, potassium, selenium, calcium

Chickpeas contain tryptophan.

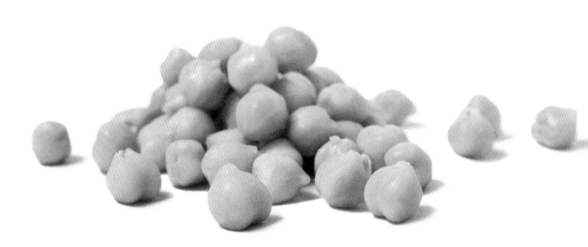

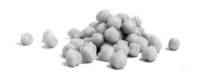

In the Middle Ages, chickpeas were ascribed many virtues, including being a diuretic and a cure for constipation and encouraging menstruation. Unfortunately, they were also criticized for causing flatulence.

VIRTUES

Reducing the risk of depression
Eating chickpeas is a quick way to increase folate intake. This vitamin promotes the secretion of dopamine, a neurotransmitter that stabilizes mood.

Predisposition to well-being
Chickpeas are a good source of vitamin B_6, which, in combination with tryptophan, promotes the secretion of serotonin. Eating chickpeas regulates not only mood, but also sleep and appetite. (See *The Chemistry of Happiness*, p. 10.)

THINGS TO REMEMBER

• To increase the body's absorption and use of iron, it is a good idea to eat chickpeas with foods that are rich in vitamin C (for instance, chickpea purée with lemon juice).

• Chickpeas in an open tin are quickly altered. Transfer them to a sealed container that you store in the refrigerator, and eat the chickpeas within two days of opening the can.

HOW TO EAT IT

Stores carry chickpea flour, also called gram flour.

Cold: in hummus or salads.

Hot: in dahls, falafel, vegetarian curry, couscous, legume loaf, soup (harira: a traditional Moroccan soup) or as a snack (baked with a drizzle of oil and spices).

CHICKPEAS AND FLATULENCE

Chickpeas are high in oligosaccharides (a sort of carbohydrate), which are responsible for flatulence. To extract as much as possible and limit the unwanted effects, drain and rinse them well after soaking. For canned chickpeas, rinse thoroughly under cold water to aid digestion and reduce the amount of sodium.

CLAMS

Composition

EXCELLENT SOURCE OF: protein, vitamins B_2 and B_{12}, zinc, copper, selenium, phosphorus

GOOD SOURCE OF: iron, vitamins A, B_3 and C, potassium

SOURCE OF: calcium

Clams contain iodine and manganese.

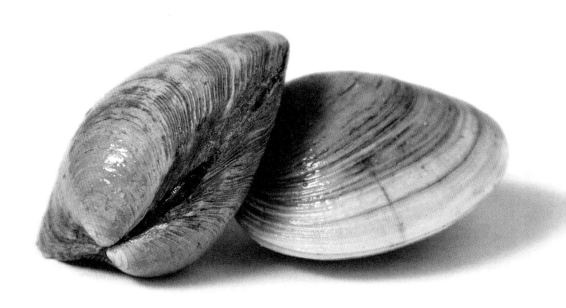

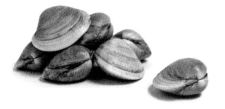

Clams have been eaten since prehistoric times, and First Nations peoples from the Atlantic Coast ate them in large quantities. In New England, in addition to being used in the famous and eponymous chowder, they were used as a tool, ornament and even currency.

VIRTUES

Reducing the risk of depression

Clams are an excellent source of vitamin B_{12}. According to a study that appeared in 2014 in *Duodecim*, insufficient intake of omega-3 and low blood levels of B_{12} increase the risk of depression.

Reducing irritability and anxiety

Clams are an excellent source of selenium, a trace element with potentially anti-depressive effects. A deficiency in food-sourced selenium is associated with irritability and anxiety, increasing the risk of depression.

THINGS TO REMEMBER

• People long believed that clams were an excellent source of iron because of an unfortunate decimal error that was perpetuated in food databases. Clams contain 2.8 g and not 28 g of iron per 100 g. So while they are not one of the best sources of iron around, they are still a good source.

• Clams are an excellent source of protein and are low in fat.

STORING AND PREPARING

• Clams should be eaten the day they are bought. Otherwise, they keep for a few days in the bottom of the refrigerator, wrapped in a moist towel.

• It is important to soak them to get rid of the sand, then wash them thoroughly before cooking.

HOW TO EAT IT

• In a cold or warm salad, in soup, chowders and sauces.

• Stuffed or marinated.

--- **DID YOU KNOW?** ---

Spring is the best season for eating fresh clams.

DARK CHOCOLATE

Composition

EXCELLENT SOURCE OF: iron, magnesium, manganese, zinc, copper

SOURCE OF: phosphorus, potassium, fiber

Chocolate contains tryptophan and theobromine.

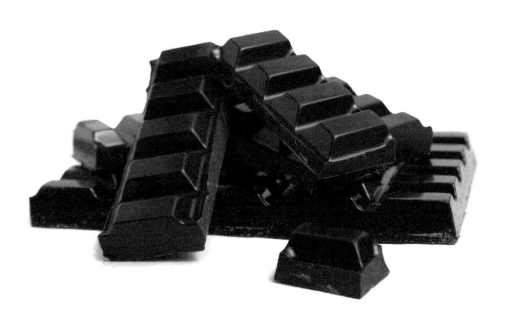

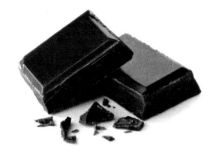

Chocolate used to be called the "food of the gods." The name of the cacao tree is Theobroma cacao (from the Greek theo, "god," and broma, "food"). The Mayans paid their taxes with cacao beans, which were used as currency at the time. These days people often say that chocolate is a natural antidepressant.

VIRTUES

Preventing depression
Cocoa includes substances that promote the production of dopamine and serotonin, two neurotransmitters associated with feelings of well-being and happiness. Plus, cocoa is one of the rare foods that contains specific substances that slow the degradation of these neurotransmitters. One study shows that eating dark chocolate can help relieve symptoms of depression, particularly among women during menopause.

Fighting chronic stress
Eating dark chocolate regularly may help mitigate symptoms of chronic stress. Daily consumption of 1½ oz (45 g) of dark chocolate for two weeks reduces blood levels of cortisol, a hormone secreted in response to chronic stress.

Improving mood
Many of the nutrients in chocolate can improve mood — and some can even create a feeling of euphoria. This is mainly due to the fat, sugar, caffeine, antioxidants, certain amino acids (such as tryptophan) and other antidepressants (such as theobromine).

THINGS TO REMEMBER

• The simple pleasure produced by the blend of flavors gives chocolate antidepressive qualities.

• Like coffee, some of the molecules in chocolate have a positive impact on cognition. It's a boost for the neurons!

• You only need to eat 1 to 1½ oz (30 to 45 g) of chocolate daily to feel the positive effects on mood.

• Choose chocolate with 70 to 85% cocoa to get the health benefits. The more cocoa the chocolate contains, the more fat it has and the less sweet it is.

• Cocoa is four to five times more antioxidizing than black tea, two to three times more antioxidizing than green tea and twice as antioxidizing as red wine.

HOW TO EAT IT

• **Bars:** one square for dessert or a few pieces in trail mix.

• **Cooked:** in a hot drink with milk and a sprinkle of cinnamon, melted, in a ganache, in mousse, in bread, muffins, chocolate croissants, as coating for fruit or almonds.

EGGS

Composition

EXCELLENT SOURCE OF: selenium, choline

GOOD SOURCE OF: vitamins B_2, B_8 and B_{12}

SOURCE OF: vitamins A, B_5, D and E, folate, phosphorus, zinc, protein

Eggs contain tryptophan and lecithin.

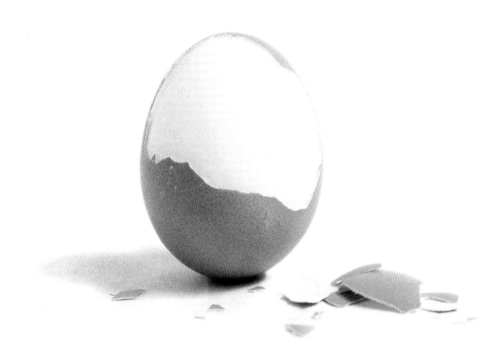

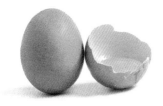

The first written record of humans eating chicken eggs dates back to 1200 BC with the Egyptians and the Chinese.

VIRTUES

Regulating mood

Eggs are an excellent source of selenium, a mineral with potentially antidepressive effects.

Reducing irritability

Vitamin B_{12} reduces irritability, mood swings and paranoia. According to a study that appeared in *Duodecim* in 2014, low blood levels of vitamin B_{12} are associated with an increased risk of depression.

Predisposition to happiness

In addition to the benefit of folate, eggs deliver the benefits of vitamins A and D, which predispose people to happiness.

THINGS TO REMEMBER

• Egg protein is complete. Eggs contain all the essential amino acids.

• Two medium eggs supply 100% of the daily recommended intake of vitamin B_{12} and about 50% of the daily recommended intake of choline.

• Watch out for salmonella, bacteria that causes food poisoning. While the risk is minimal, only eat raw or undercooked eggs (for example, in mayonnaise, egg vinaigrette or in a mousse for dessert) if you are sure they are fresh and pasteurized. The inside of the egg must not come in contact with the outside of the shell to avoid any risk of contamination.

STORING

To properly store eggs, keep them on a shelf in the refrigerator and not on the door, preferably in their box so that you know the expiry date. Eggs should be placed tips down. They will keep this way for about three weeks. To find out whether an egg is fresh, dunk it in a saucepan of water. If it sinks, it's fresh; if it floats, it's too old to eat.

HOW TO EAT IT

• Poached, hard-boiled, scrambled, sunny side up, in salads and in sandwiches.

• In omelets, frittatas, soufflés, quiches, crêpes and cakes.

• For making pasta and binding sauces.

─────── **DID YOU KNOW?** ───────

The color of the shell (white or brown) has no bearing on the nutritional value of eggs and depends exclusively on the type of chicken.

LENTILS

Composition

EXCELLENT SOURCE OF: iron, folate, phosphorus, copper, protein

GOOD SOURCE OF: manganese, fiber

SOURCE OF: vitamins B_1, B_2, B_3, B_5 and B_6, magnesium, potassium, zinc, selenium

Lentils contain tryptophan and tyrosine.

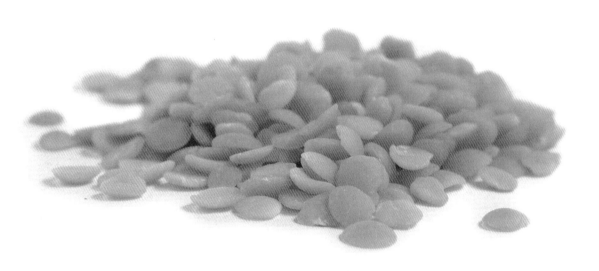

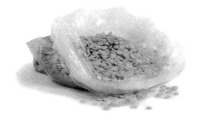

Lentils are a dried legume, like chickpeas and dried beans (for instance, white and red). They are one of the easiest foods to digest and one of the most nutritious.

VIRTUES

Reducing mood disorders

A folate deficiency may be associated with depression and mood disorders. Eating 1 cup (250 ml) of cooked lentils meets 90% of the recommended daily intake of folate.

Greater sense of well-being

Rich in protein, carbohydrates and vitamins, lentils are the ultimate filling, comfort food. They are a good source of tryptophan, an amino acid that, in synergy with B vitamins, is transformed into serotonin by the body. Also called the "happiness hormone," serotonin regulates sleep, appetite and mood.

Stabilizing mood

Lentils are rich in tyrosine, an amino acid that is essential to synthesizing a number of neurotransmitters (including dopamine) involved in stabilizing mood. (See *The Chemistry of Happiness*, p. 10.)

THINGS TO REMEMBER

• To promote the body's absorption and use of iron and tryptophan, you should round out a plate of lentils with a source of vitamin C.

• Lentils are one of the easiest legumes to digest. They are a good source of plant protein, provided they are combined with a grain (for instance, wheat, barley, millet or rice) and nuts, because they are missing an essential amino acid, methionine. Eat two thirds grains and one third dried legumes, such as lentils. Children, teens, the elderly and pregnant women should eat them in the same meal, but other people can spread them out over the day.

• Adding baking soda to the soaking water (¼ tsp per 4 cups/1 liter of water) reduces soaking and cooking time. However, baking soda destroys the vitamin B_1 present in legumes and gives them a pasty texture.

HOW TO EAT IT

• In dahls, soups, vegetarian stews (made with vegetables and rice), salads, veggie burgers or as a meat substitute in shepherd's pie.

• As a side for salmon, veal shanks or braised pork.

─────── **DID YOU KNOW?** ───────

Nutritionally speaking, there is no significant difference between red and green lentils.

PINTO BEANS

Composition

EXCELLENT SOURCE OF: fiber, protein, vitamin B_1, folate, manganese, copper, iron

GOOD SOURCE OF: vitamin B_6, magnesium, potassium, selenium, zinc, phosphorus, calcium

SOURCE OF: vitamins B_2 and B_5

Pinto beans contain omega-3 fatty acids.

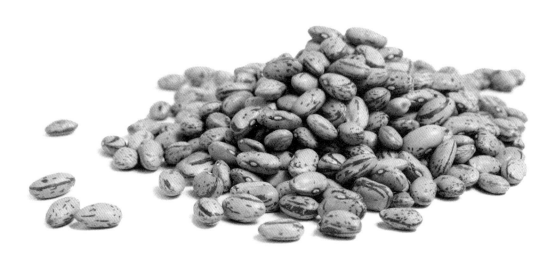

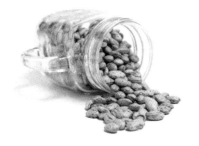

The bean's spotted appearance is what earned it the name *pinto*, which means "painted" in Spanish.

VIRTUES

Providing support for antidepressants
According to an article in the *American Journal of Psychiatry*, certain people who suffered from serious depression but were not responding very well to their treatment saw their symptoms diminish when their antidepressant was combined with folate supplements.

Restoring energy and morale
Pinto beans are a good source of protein, vitamins and nutrients. These nutrients (including magnesium, zinc and B complex vitamins) are essential to maintaining the chemical balance of the brain. A deficiency in nutrients could create a drop in morale.

Combating stress
Chronic or acute stress can lead to depression when the body does not have enough magnesium to meet its needs. Eating pinto beans combats fatigue, irritability, memory problems and confusion.

THINGS TO REMEMBER

• People who eat little or no animal protein may benefit from combining legumes with grains or nuts to get complete proteins (with all the essential amino acids). These combinations should occur in the same meal for children, teens, the elderly and pregnant women, but can be spread out over the day for anyone else.

• Pinto beans can substitute for red beans in most recipes.

SOAKING

If you buy dried beans, it is important to soak them overnight in the refrigerator, replace the soaking water once or twice, cook them thoroughly and rinse them well after cooking. If flatulence is a problem, choose a quick soaking method (see *Pinto Beans and Flatulance*, p. 169).

HOW TO EAT IT

• Puréed (with garlic, onion and chili powder) to make a spread or for sandwiches.

• In a bean salad, soup, chili or bean loaf.

———— SOMETHING TO DISCOVER ————

In Mexico, it is traditional to cook pinto beans for a long time in slightly sweet water, and to let them sit overnight before frying. Grated cheese, hot peppers, roasted peanuts, onions, green and red peppers and spices (ginger, garlic, cumin, coriander seeds and others) are added to them. They are served in tortillas.

PUMPKIN SEEDS

Composition

EXCELLENT SOURCE OF: protein, magnesium, copper, phosphorus, manganese, iron

GOOD SOURCE OF: zinc

SOURCE OF: vitamin B_1, selenium, potassium

Pumpkin seeds contain tryptophan, tyrosine and phenylalanine.

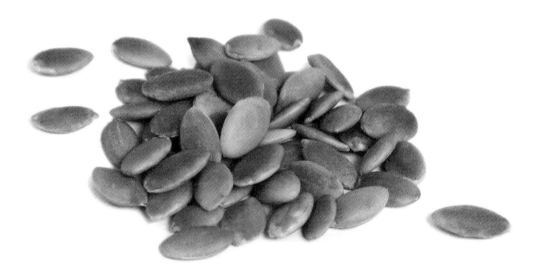

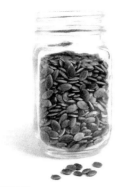

A number of First Nations, including the Menominee and Algonquin, thought pumpkin seeds to be a diuretic. They were also used as a dewormer (crushed with honey, water or milk) by North American colonists.

VIRTUES

Reducing anxiety
Pumpkin seeds are an excellent source of manganese, an essential trace element that helps fight anxiety. Regular consumption of food rich in magnesium (such as pumpkin seeds) also helps fight fatigue, irritability, memory problems and confusion, promoting a sense of calm and a state of relaxation.

Stabilizing mood
Pumpkin seeds contain tyrosine and phenylalanine, two amino acids that go into making dopamine, a neurotransmitter that regulates mood and motivation.

Support in treating depression
According to an article published in the *British Journal of Psychiatry*, pumpkin seeds contain tryptophan and could therefore reinforce the treatment of light-to-moderate depression.

THINGS TO REMEMBER
• To benefit from the virtues of pumpkin seeds, it is better to eat them raw or dried rather than roasted.

• By weight, pumpkin seeds have more iron than liver. Not only does iron improve vitality and stimulate the immune system, it also helps synthesize certain hormones and regulates the secretion of certain neurotransmitters. To better absorb the iron, it is a good idea to consume foods rich in vitamin C (such as pepper, tomato, strawberries and citrus).

STORING
Pumpkin seeds go rancid quite easily, so it's a good idea to keep them in the refrigerator.

HOW TO EAT IT
• Plain or dried, as a snack, in salads or on cereal.

• In muffins, granola bars, hamburgers or spreads.

—— PREPARING SEEDS AT HOME ——
When you cook fresh pumpkin, carefully wash the seeds and pat them dry, then spread them on a baking sheet. Spray with oil and season to taste. Then bake them at 350°F (180°C) for 20 minutes.

RED GRAPES

Composition

GOOD SOURCE OF: vitamin K, manganese
SOURCE OF: copper, vitamins B_1, B_6 and C, potassium
Red grapes contain resveratrol.

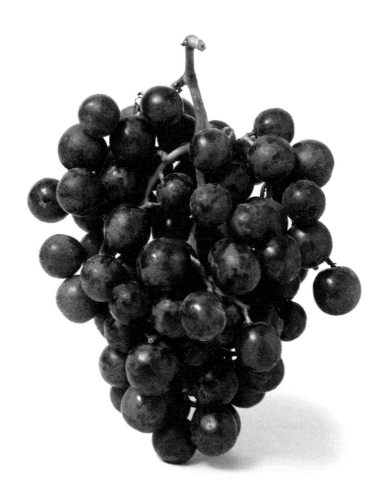

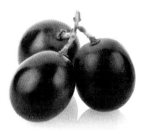

Since ancient times, grapes have been ascribed many virtues. They were considered a miracle remedy for constipation, gout, arthritis and skin problems.

VIRTUES

Mitigating symptoms of depression
A number of studies suggest that the resveratrol in grapes could reduce depressive type symptoms and have therapeutic potential in the treatment of serious depression. Exactly how it does this is not yet fully understood, but there are many avenues for research.

Encouraging well-being
Red grapes are a source of vitamin C. Not only does this antioxidant vitamin strengthen the immune system, it also helps in the synthesis of neurotransmitters, particularly serotonin.

Stabilizing mood
Manganese, which red grapes are an excellent source of, limits mood swings.

THINGS TO REMEMBER
• Red grapes have twice the antioxidant power as green grapes, because of the higher amount of antioxidants in their bright color.

• Other benefits: red grapes are an effective ally in the fight against aging (particularly skin aging) and cancer.

• To enjoy the benefits of grapes, they can be consumed in the form of juice or wine (in moderation).

HOW TO EAT IT
• On a cheese plate or in a salad.

• In juice, whole in a fruit salad, as a topping for cake, waffles or pancakes, in a jelly or jam.

———— CHOOSING GRAPES ————

Choose nice full bunches (the grapes must not detach easily from the stem). Grapes need to be rinsed thoroughly before eating.

RED ONIONS

Composition

SOURCE OF: folate, fiber, vitamins B$_6$ and C, manganese, potassium

Red onion contains quercetin.

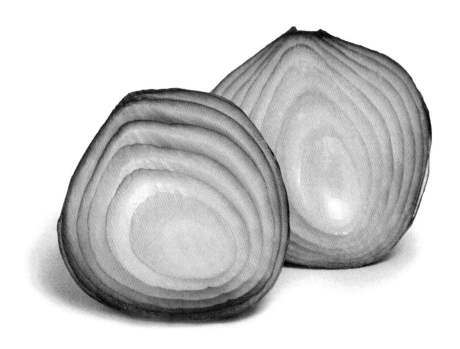

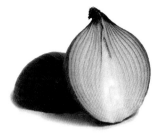

Onions are one of the earliest vegetables consumed by humans. From way back, oignons were believed to have all sorts of medicinal properties, from reducing baldness to curing infections and fighting cellulite.

VIRTUES

Preventing depression
Eaten regularly, red onions increase intake of vitamin B_6 and folate. People suffering from depression often do not get enough of these vitamins.

Reducing anxiety
Researchers have shown that quercetin, an antioxidant found in onions, could have an effect on anxiety.

THINGS TO REMEMBER
Red onion is much richer in antioxidants than paler onions. Cooked onion is richer in antioxidants than raw onion. Antioxidants protect the body's cells from the damage caused by free radicals, responsible for premature aging.

STORING
• It's best to store onions in a cool, dry place, away from light.

• Don't leave cut onions out. Not only do they lose a large proportion of their vitamins and minerals, but they can also become harmful because of oxidation. Cut them in rings and freeze them until ready to use.

HOW TO EAT IT
Raw: in salads and on hamburgers.

Cooked: confit, sautéed with vegetables, in soups and quiches and on pizza.

———— DID YOU KNOW? ————

To avoid irritated eyes, rinse onions under water after peeling, because the molecule responsible for tears (syn-Propanethial-S-oxide) is highly water soluble.

SALMON

Composition

EXCELLENT SOURCE OF: omega-3 fatty acids, protein,
phosphorus, selenium, vitamins B_1, B_3, B_5, B_6, B_{12} and D
GOOD SOURCE OF: potassium
SOURCE OF: magnesium, zinc, copper, folate, vitamin B_2, iron

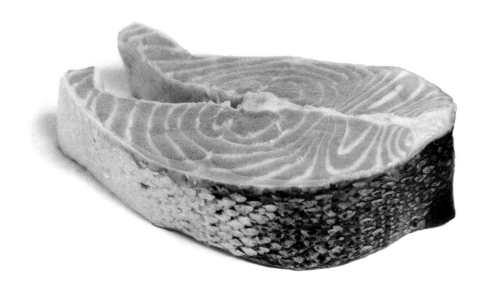

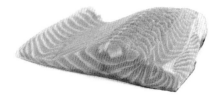

The term *salmon* (Latin in origin for "to leap") refers to several species of fish that belong to the Salmonidae family. These ocean or freshwater fish live mainly in the northern Atlantic and Pacific oceans. The salmon found on the market is largely farmed.

VIRTUES

Preventing depression
Studies show that people who eat fish rich in omega-3 fatty acids (such as salmon) at least once a week have a lower risk of depression.

Improving well-being
Salmon's high content of vitamins B_1, B_6, B_{12} and D make it the perfect food for fighting symptoms of depression. Regular consumption helps regulate sleep, appetite and mood.

Reducing irritability
Salmon is an excellent source of selenium, a deficiency that is associated with irritability and anxiety. A 2½ oz (75 g) portion of cooked salmon meets about 70% of the daily recommended intake of selenium.

THINGS TO REMEMBER

• Salmon is one of the best sources of omega-3 fatty acids, which reduce the risk of cardiovascular disease. However, the quantity depends on the species; Atlantic salmon has higher levels.

• Eating the bones from canned fish (carefully) increases calcium intake.

COOKING

• Omega-3s, like those contained in fatty fish, are thermolabile fatty acids, which means that they are very sensitive to heat and quickly degrade when exposed to high temperatures. To benefit from the omega-3s, choose gentle and fast cooking methods (steamed or en papillote, for example).

• It is also a good idea to cook fish without adding any fat. The main nutrients in fish (omega-3s, vitamins A, D and E) are liposoluble, which means that are soluble in fat. This means that if the fish is cooked in contact with oil, the nutrients leach from the fish to the fat.

HOW TO EAT IT

Raw: gravlax, tartare, ceviche or sashimi.

Cooked: steamed, en papillote, grilled, poached or smoked.

SALMON: RAW OR COOKED?

Raw fish delivers the same nutrients as cooked fish, provided it is cooked gently and with no fat. Raw fish is not recommended for young children, pregnant women, the elderly or people with a compromised immune system.

SARDINES

Composition

EXCELLENT SOURCE OF: protein, omega-3 fatty acids, calcium, selenium, vitamins B_3, B_{12} and D, phosphorus

GOOD SOURCE OF: iron, copper, vitamin B_2

SOURCE OF: zinc, potassium

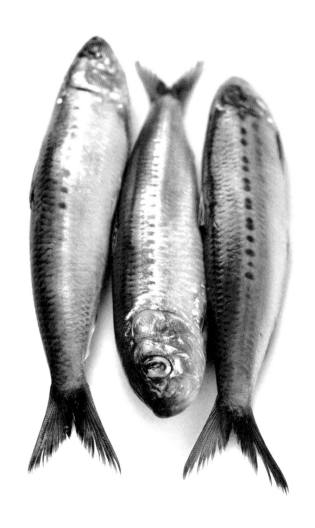

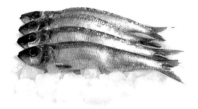

The word *sardine* comes from the Latin *Sardae sine sardinae*, which means "fish of Sardinia." Fished since time immemorial in the Mediterranean, they are a staple in the diet of Italians and Portuguese. The word *sardine* refers to not just one fish, but some 20 varieties of small fish.

VIRTUES

Reducing the risk of depression

Eating 3 to 4 oz (about 90 to 120 g) of fish rich in omega-3 fatty acids daily, such as sardines, could reduce the risk of mental health disorders, particularly depression.

Fighting seasonal affective disorder

Foods rich in vitamin D stimulate the production of serotonin, a neurotransmitter that regulates sleep, appetite and mood. (See *The Chemistry of Happiness*, p. 10)

THINGS TO REMEMBER

• Sardines are an excellent source of complete protein. They contain all of the essential amino acids the body needs.

• Cooking sardines en papillote preserves the omega-3s.

• Eating the bones in canned sardines (carefully) increases calcium intake.

HOW TO EAT IT

Fresh: grilled, in bouillabaisse or as tapas.

Canned: on canapés or in salad.

———— DID YOU KNOW? ————

Small fish such as sardines contain fewer pollutants, such as mercury, than large ones, because they don't store heavy metals.

SPINACH

Composition

EXCELLENT SOURCE OF: vitamins A and K, folate
SOURCE OF: vitamins C and E, magnesium, manganese, iron, potassium
Spinach contains betaine.

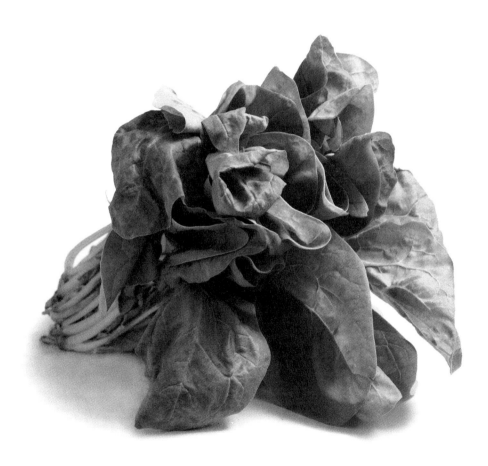

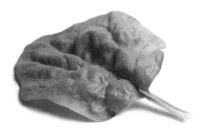

In cooking, the term *Florentine* means a dish in which the main ingredient (often eggs or fish) is served on a bed of braised spinach. We owe the appellation to Catherine de Medici, the queen of France, born in Florence, Italy. She is said to have liked spinach so much that she insisted her cooks travel with her to prepare her favorite dishes.

VIRTUES

Stabilizing mood
Eating spinach promotes the natural secretion of dopamine and serotonin (see *The Chemistry of Happiness*, p. 10) in the body because of its high content of betaine, a compound with potentially antidepressive effects.

Reducing symptoms of depression
Spinach is an excellent source of folate. It has been shown that people who suffer from depression often have abnormally low folate levels. Eating spinach regularly may mitigate the symptoms of depression.

Promoting relaxation
Regularly eating foods with a significant amount of magnesium (such as spinach) apparently promotes relaxation and restorative sleep.

THINGS TO REMEMBER

Spinach is more nutritious cooked than raw. In equal portions, cooked spinach contains about six times as much lutein, zeaxanthin and betaine than raw. Boiled spinach is also a better source of vitamins and minerals than raw. But it is a good idea to eat spinach both cooked and raw to get the benefits of its vitamin C and folate, which is heat sensitive.

HOW TO EAT IT

Raw: in salad, smoothies or sandwiches.

Cooked: in soup, lasagna, omelets, quiche, as stuffing for fish or chicken, in gratins or dips.

———— COMMON MISCONCEPTIONS ————
Spinach is high in iron.
FALSE. Spinach has long been touted as being high in iron. The idea, promulgated by Popeye, is the result of a decimal error. At the end of the 19th century, a chemist established the composition of spinach. When recopying the iron content, the decimal point was shifted to the right. It took until the 1930s for researchers to correct the error. But it was too late: Popeye and his spinach had made it around the world! What's more, plant-sourced iron is less easily assimilated by the body than iron from animal sources.

SUNFLOWER SEEDS

Composition

EXCELLENT SOURCE OF: vitamins B_5 and E, folate, manganese, phosphorus, copper, selenium

GOOD SOURCE OF: vitamin B_6, magnesium, iron, fiber

SOURCE OF: protein, vitamins B_1, B_2 and B_3, potassium

Sunflower seeds contain tryptophan.

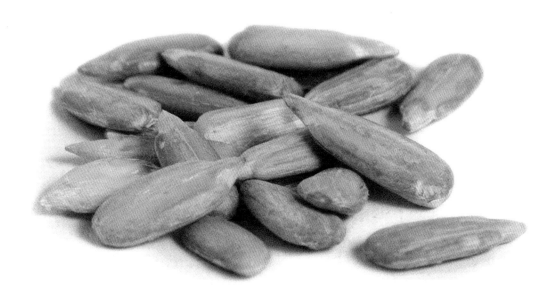

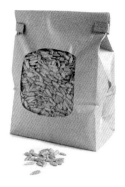

Sunflower seeds have long been considered a natural antidepressant. The Ukraine and Russia are two of the largest producers of sunflower seeds.

VIRTUES

Reducing the risk of depression
Eating sunflower seeds increases your folate intake, which promotes the secretion of dopamine. Studies suggest that eating food rich in folate could reduce the risk of depression.

Encouraging well-being
Eating sunflower seeds could have a positive impact on mood, appetite and sleep, because they provide the body with tryptophan (an amino acid) and several vitamins that combined promote the secretion of serotonin (see *The Chemistry of Happiness*, p. 10).

Reducing mood disorders
A small-scale study showed that large quantities of selenium could improve mood in patients who suffer from mild to moderate depression. Plus a selenium deficiency could exacerbate mood disorders, particularly among people who suffer from hypothyroidism, which is inadequate functioning of the thyroid gland.

THINGS TO REMEMBER
Unsaturated fat accounts for about 90% of the fat in sunflower seeds. This fat seems to reduce the risk of depression.

STORING
To store sunflower seeds and prevent them from going rancid quickly, you can refrigerate them, or freeze them for even longer storage.

HOW TO EAT IT
• Plain for a nutritious snack (also with dried fruits in trail mix), in salads and cereals, crushed into nut butter or in pesto.

• In muffins, granola bars, bread or stuffing.

─────── **DID YOU KNOW?** ───────

The name of the sunflower is often said to come from the fact that the flower turns toward the sun, but this is a myth. The growing stem does follow the movement of the sun, but once it reaches maturity and is flowering, it is insensitive to light.

SWEET POTATO

Composition

EXCELLENT SOURCE OF: vitamin A, manganese, copper

GOOD SOURCE OF: fiber, vitamins B_6 and C, potassium

SOURCE OF: vitamins B_2 and B_5, magnesium, phosphorus, iron

Sweet potatoes contain tryptophan.

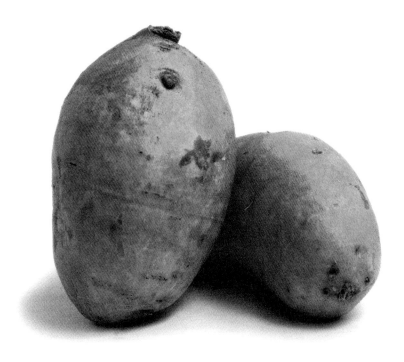

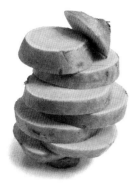

Sweet potatoes are tubers but are not in the same family as the potato. They are sweeter than potatoes and contain twice as much fiber.

VIRTUES

Stabilizing mood
Sweet potatoes are rich in manganese, making them the perfect ally for proper brain functioning. A medium-sized sweet potato provides about 50% of the daily recommended intake of manganese.

Predisposition to happiness
Sweet potatoes are a good source of vitamin B_6, which, along with tryptophan, promotes the secretion of serotonin. Eating this tuber could therefore regulate not only mood, but also sleep and appetite (see *The Chemistry of Happiness*, p. 10).

THINGS TO REMEMBER
There are over 400 varieties of white, yellow, orange and purple sweet potatoes. The varieties with orange and purple flesh are more nutritious.

STORING
Sweet potatoes should be stored in a cool place, but not in the refrigerator. If you store them at under 50°F (10°C), they get hard and lose their flavor. If they show signs of mold, throw them away.

HOW TO EAT IT
Sweet potatoes are cooked and prepared like potatoes or winter squash. They can replace them in recipes.

Savory: boiled, puréed, baked unpeeled in the oven (en papillote or as fries), fried (chips or fries), in soups, salads, croquettes, soufflés, frittatas, couscous or curries.

Sweet: in flans, creams, cakes, cookies, muffins, white cheese verrines or flambéed with rum.

—— DID YOU KNOW? ——

Sweet potatoes are a staple in many countries of Asia, Africa and Latin America, as well as in the southern United States.

WALNUTS

Composition

EXCELLENT SOURCE OF: manganese

GOOD SOURCE OF: copper, magnesium

SOURCE OF: protein, vitamins B_1, B_3 and B_6, folate, zinc, phosphorus, iron, fiber

Walnuts contain omega-3 fatty acids and are a good source of tryptophan.

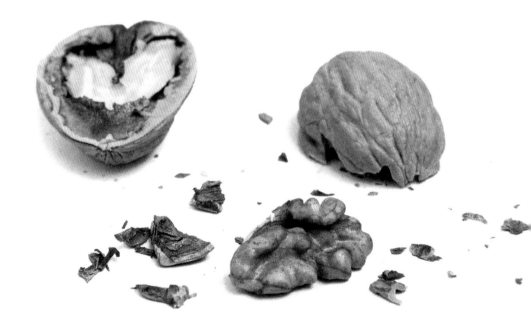

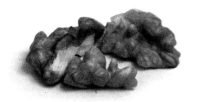

The Latin name for the walnut tree, *Juglans*, is a contraction of *Jovis* and *glans*, which means "the gland of Jupiter," referring to the Roman belief that the highly fertile walnut tree had been given to them by Jupiter.

VIRTUES

Promoting happiness

According to a clinical study that appeared in the *Journal of Proteome Research*, people who ate 1 oz (30 g) of nuts (including walnuts) daily for 12 weeks secreted more serotonin, the "happiness hormone," than those who did not. According to a number of studies, eating plenty of foods that are rich in vitamin B_6 and tryptophan promotes the synthesis of serotonin.

Reducing anxiety

Generally speaking, food that contains significant amounts of B vitamins reduces anxiety, stress and even depression. According to researchers in Maryland, a deficiency, particularly in vitamin B_6 (which walnuts are a source of), is associated with depression.

THINGS TO REMEMBER

• Walnuts are 70% polyunsaturated fats. Their balance between omega-6 and omega-3 fatty acids is optimal for health.

• Other benefits: according to a number of studies, eating walnuts regularly (5 portions of ¼ cup/60 ml per week) lowers total cholesterol and LDL cholesterol (bad cholesterol) and even slightly increases HDL cholesterol (good cholesterol).

STORING

Walnuts oxidize and go rancid quickly. It is better to buy them in the shell because it protects them from air and light. Keep them in an airtight jar away from light, in the refrigerator or the freezer.

HOW TO EAT IT

• As a snack, plain or roasted, in trail mix with dried fruit.

• In Waldorf or endive salads, bowls of cereal, yogurt, granola and granola bars.

• In tapenade, stuffing, bread, pasta sauce or on a cheese plate.

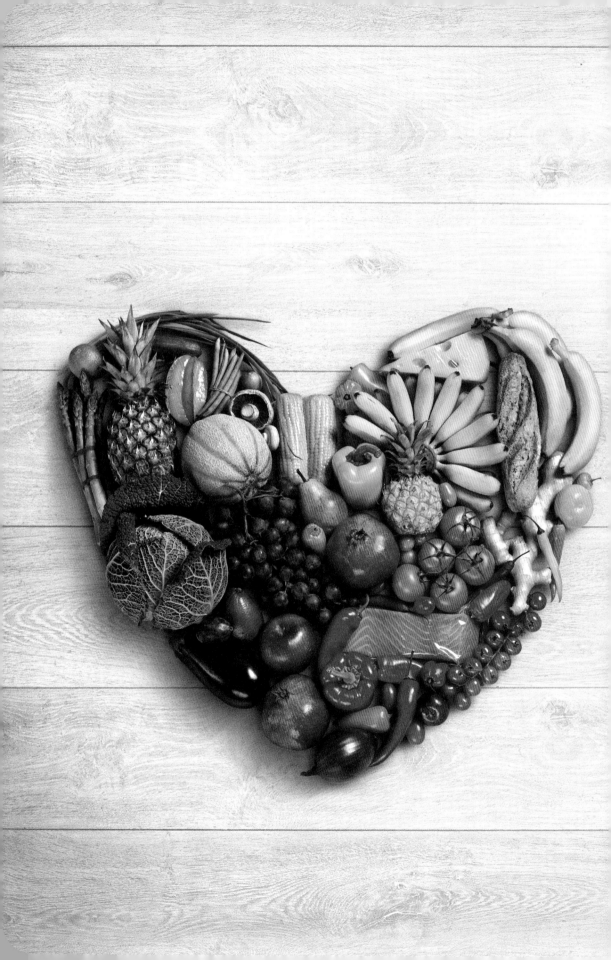

FACT OR FICTION

YOU SHOULD ONLY EAT ORGANIC FRUITS AND VEGETABLES.

FALSE.

According to a number of studies, organic fruits and vegetables have more antioxidants (although sometimes marginally more) than regular ones. They are not treated with pesticides or fungicides, so the plants naturally produce more of these nutrients to protect against attack.

Every year, in the United States, the Environmental Working Group studies the amount of pesticide residue in some 40 fruits and vegetables. For food with the least residue, you do not absolutely need to buy organic. But it is a good idea to choose organic products for food that does contain the most residue. (See table below.)

If you don't eat organic food, you should still eat fruits and vegetables from traditional agriculture rather than eliminating them from your diet. Pesticides are much less of a health risk than deficiencies in fiber, vitamins, minerals and phytonutrients from a diet that doesn't include many fruits and vegetables. The risk of pesticide residue is negligible compared with the health benefits of a diet with plenty of fruits and vegetables.

CLEAN 15	DIRTY DOZEN
Asparagus	Apples
Avocados	Celery
Cabbage	Cherry tomatoes
Cantaloupe	Chile peppers
Cauliflower	Cucumber
Corn	Grapes
Eggplant	Nectarines
Grapefruit	Peaches
Kiwi	Potatoes
Mango	Red peppers
Onions	Spinach
Papaya	Strawberries
Peas	
Pineapple	
Sweet potato	

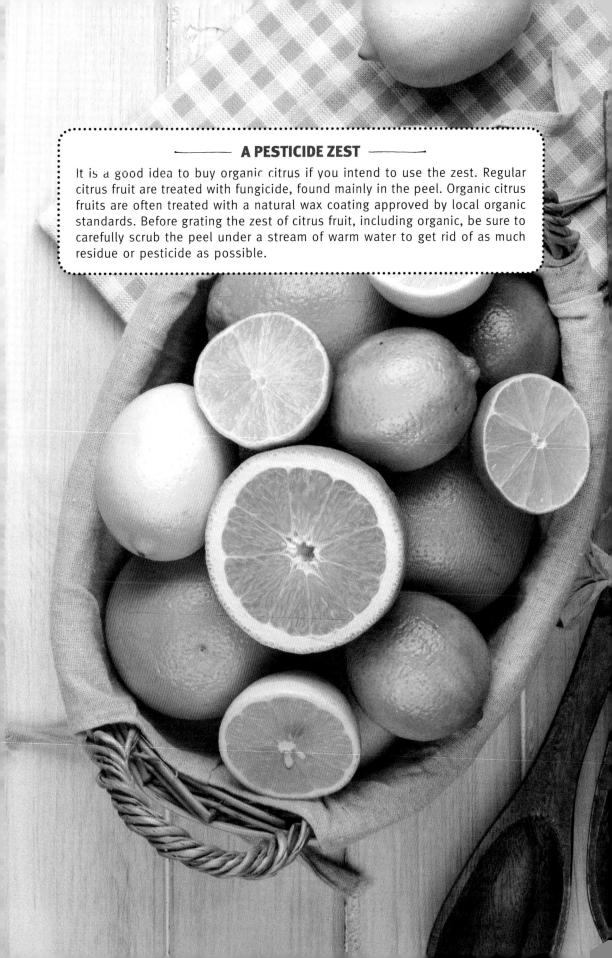

A PESTICIDE ZEST

It is a good idea to buy organic citrus if you intend to use the zest. Regular citrus fruit are treated with fungicide, found mainly in the peel. Organic citrus fruits are often treated with a natural wax coating approved by local organic standards. Before grating the zest of citrus fruit, including organic, be sure to carefully scrub the peel under a stream of warm water to get rid of as much residue or pesticide as possible.

FRESH VEGETABLES ARE MORE NUTRITIOUS THAN FROZEN.

FALSE.

Contrary to popular belief, fresh vegetables are not necessarily more nutritious than frozen.

Generally, the fresher the food, the more nutritious it is, because vitamins and minerals are sensitive to light, oxygen and heat. Fruits and vegetables should be eaten as soon as possible after they are picked.

Fresh vegetables: When vegetables are bought fresh from the market or the grocery store, they may have spent a long time in transport and storage and therefore lose a significant amount of nutrients.

Frozen vegetables: Fresh vegetables destined for freezing are processed a few hours after being picked. The storage time is very short, preserving their nutrients. The vegetables are blanched (dipped in boiling water) before being frozen, a process that reduces their content of water-soluble vitamins (in particular, vitamins B_1 and C) and certain antioxidants. However, other nutrients (such as water-soluble vitamins A and E) are better preserved, so frozen vegetables contain more than fresh vegetables.

Whether fresh or frozen, all vegetables are good sources of nutrients and fiber. Variety is the healthiest bet.

FROZEN PRODUCTS: A FEW PRECAUTIONS ...

Frozen products should be defrosted in the refrigerator and not at room temperature. Ideally, they should be consumed within 24 hours. Never refreeze a defrosted product, because the bacteria that develop when defrosting can cause food poisoning. Plus, defrosting changes taste and texture. Once cooked, frozen vegetables can be kept as long as fresh vegetables.

PRE-CUT VEGETABLES AREN'T NUTRITIOUS.

FALSE.

Luckily for busy people, the vitamin and mineral content of pre-cut vegetables is still pretty good. Of course, they are less rich in vitamin C and folate than whole fresh vegetables, but still a considerable amount remains. For example, women need 75 mg of vitamin C per day. Even if the content of vitamin C in a green pepper is reduced 20% when it is pre-cut, it will still meet 95% of her needs. Plus, it won't be the only source of vitamin C during the day.

So don't be afraid to make life easier for yourself. The important thing with vegetables is to eat them.

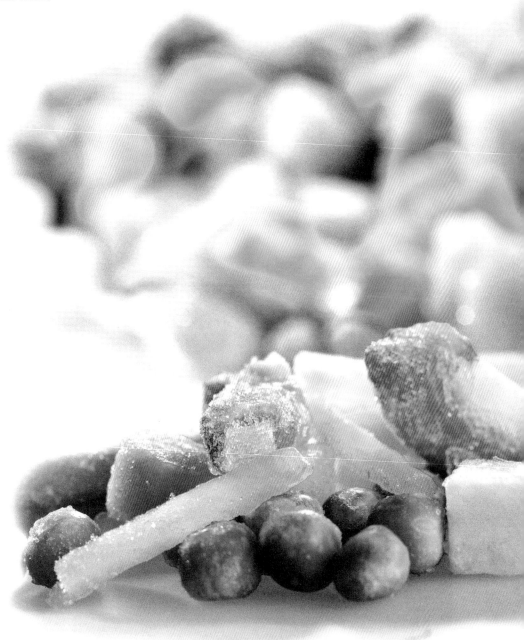

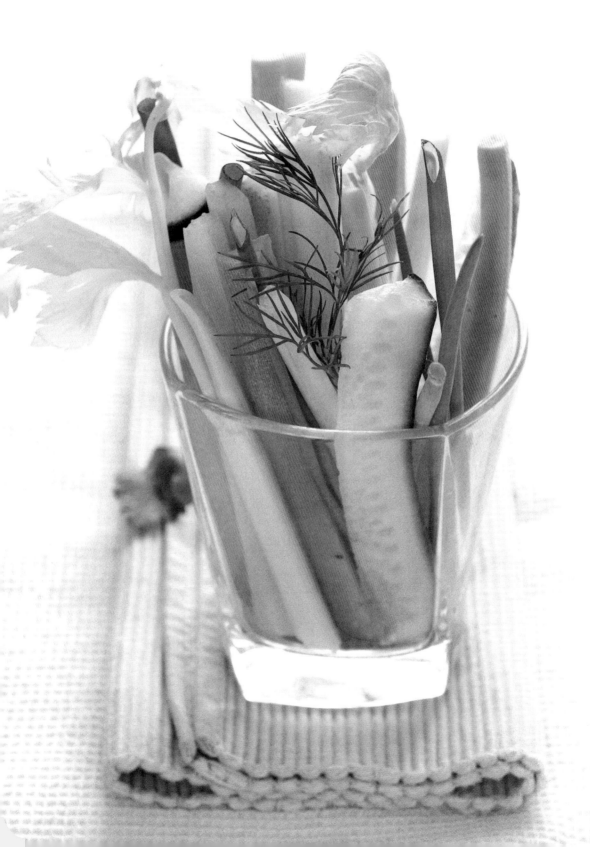

IT'S BETTER TO EAT FRUITS AND VEGETABLES WHEN MATURE.

TRUE.

With few exceptions, fruits and vegetables pack more nutrition when mature (however, broccoli sprouts are richer in antioxidants than mature broccoli). They become richer in vitamins and minerals as they mature, and many of the beneficial compounds are found in the pigment that gives them their color. However, the amount of nutrients depends on many other factors (e.g., sun, heat, soil, etc.). Taste is at its peak when products are consumed at maturity.

COOKING REDUCES THE NUTRITIONAL VALUE OF FOOD.

FALSE, BUT . . .

Cooking too long can reduce the content of vitamins in foods, and some of the minerals can leach into the cooking water. So it is a good idea to cook vegetables as quickly as possible and serve them right away, and to limit the amount of cooking water. Sautéing, steaming and baking are the ideal cooking methods for preserving nutrients. Some foods, such as orange vegetables (carrots, sweet potatoes, etc.) and tomatoes, contain more antioxidants after cooking. For instance, according to certain studies, the amount of lycopene (an antioxidant) in tomatoes doubles after 30 minutes of cooking. And don't forget that cooking destroys unwanted bacteria in certain foods and makes them easier to digest.

Studies show that microwave and steam cooking preserve the most nutrients in vegetables. Since raw food delivers more vitamins and helps control weight because it is more filling, it should be on the menu more often. But don't forget that a balanced diet is primarily a varied diet.

NUTRITIONALLY SPEAKING, CANNED FISH HAS ALL THE BENEFITS OF FRESH FISH.

TRUE.

This is true provided the fish isn't soaking in oil. A portion of canned fish can replace a portion of fresh fish, and deliver savings. Neither canning nor freezing alters the nutrients found in fish. Sardines, mackerel, salmon, tuna and other fish can be eaten fresh, canned or frozen.

TIPS FOR PRESERVING
──── VITAMINS AND NUTRIENTS ────

- Eat fruits and vegetables soon after buying or picking them. The longer they are stored, the more nutrients they lose.

- Wash whole vegetables and don't let them soak, to limit the loss of water-soluble vitamins (see table below).

- Preferably, don't cut fruits and vegetables too much in advance because many vitamins are sensitive to oxygen and light.

- Limit cooking time for vegetables (serve them crunchy) to preserve heat-sensitive nutrients. Exceptions: lycopene, found in tomatoes, and quercetin, found in onions. These two antioxidants are not broken down by heat; in fact they are more easily assimilated after cooking.

- Ideally, steam vegetables to prevent water-soluble vitamins from leaching into the cooking water.

- To preserve fat-soluble vitamins (see table below), which are not highly water soluble, braise, steam or boil.

- When cooking in water, bring the water to a boil and then add the vegetables (except for potatoes, which are added to cold water).

- Avoid frying or cooking at high temperatures, because this produces potentially carcinogenic, toxic compounds.

WATER-SOLUBLE VITAMINS	FAT-SOLUBLE VITAMINS
B complex vitamins	Vitamin A
Vitamin C	Vitamin D
	Vitamin E
	Vitamin K

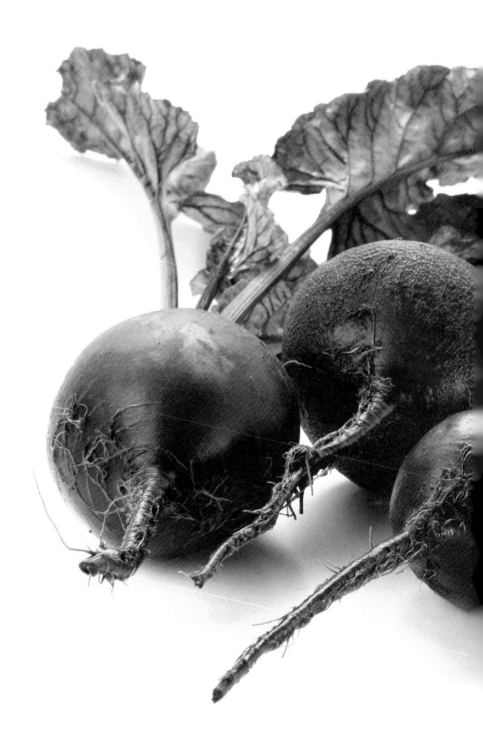

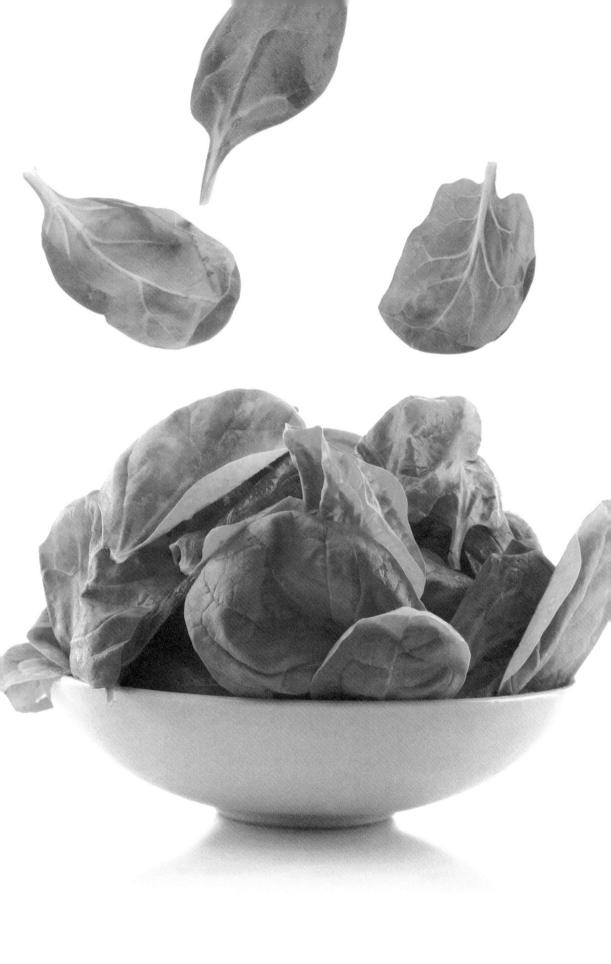

RECIPES

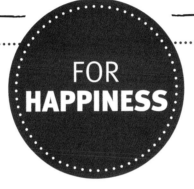

FOR HAPPINESS

LEGEND

🥣 Preparation   🥄 Soaking

❄️ Refrigeration   🍲 Cooking

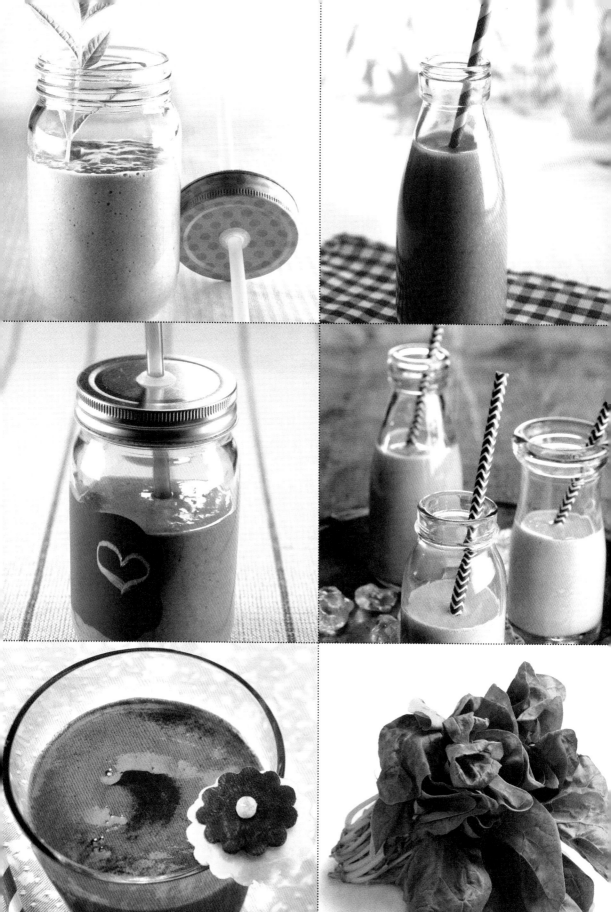

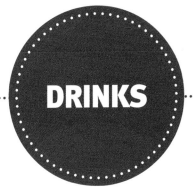

DRINKS

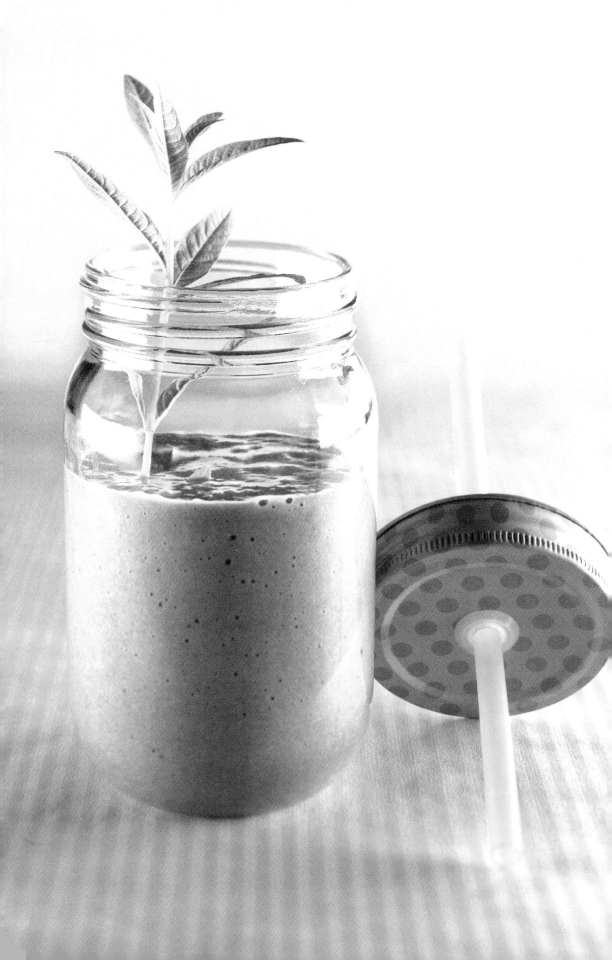

SPINACH BANANA
SMOOTHIE

2 SERVINGS
5 MINUTES

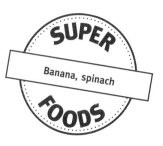

Banana, spinach

INGREDIENTS

2 cups (500 ml) almond milk

½ cup (125 ml) plain
Greek yogurt

2 cups (500 ml) roughly torn
spinach

1 cup (250 ml) roughly torn
kale, without stems

1 ripe **banana**, in pieces

1 tbsp almond butter

1 tbsp chia seeds

4 fresh mint leaves

METHOD

In a blender or food processor, combine all ingredients and blend for 20 to 35 seconds or until smooth.

Add water or almond milk as needed for a smoother consistency.

Nutrition Facts Per serving	
Amount	% Daily Value
Calories 150	
Fat 1.5 g	2%
Saturated 0.3 g	
+ Trans 0 g	
Polyunsaturated 0.5 g	
Omega-6 0.3 g	
Omega-3 0.4 g	
Monounsaturated 0.1 g	
Cholesterol 2 mg	0%
Sodium 110 mg	4%
Potassium 250 mg	7%
Carbohydrates 16 g	5%
Fiber 6 g	24%
Sugar 8 g	
Protein 18 g	
Vitamin A 20 ER	2%
Vitamin C 20 mg	35%
Calcium 185 mg	15%
Iron 0.8 mg	6%
Phosphorus 51 mg	4%

DID YOU KNOW?

If you keep bananas with other fruit in a basket or, even better, in a brown paper bag, they will make everything ripen faster because of ethylene, a gas they give off as they ripen.

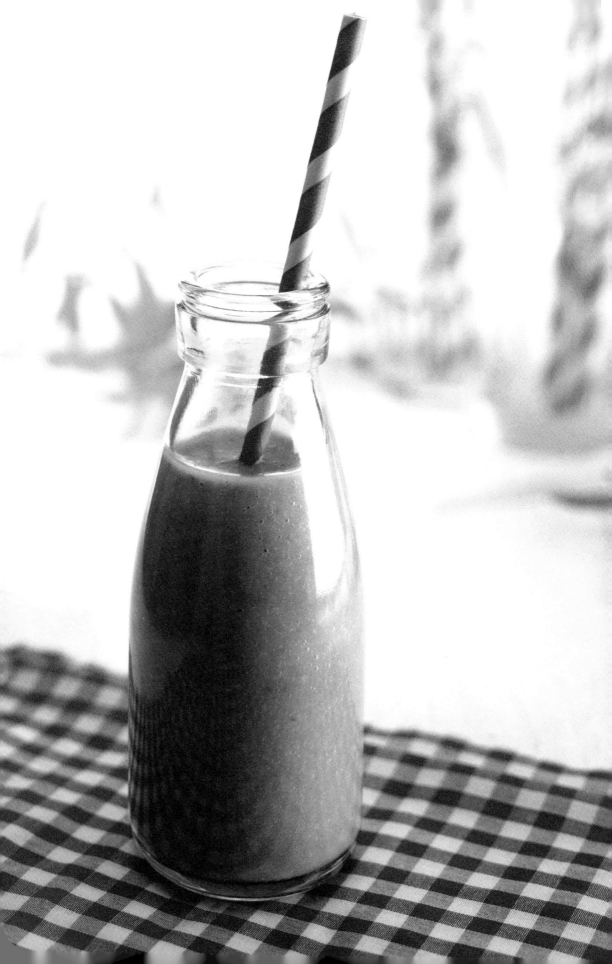

GOOD MORNING
SMOOTHIE

2 SERVINGS
5 MINUTES

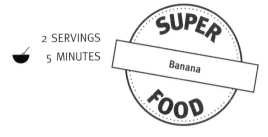

SUPER
Banana
FOOD

INGREDIENTS

2 cups (500 ml) almond milk

½ cup (125 ml) plain
Greek yogurt

1 cup (250 ml) fresh or
frozen raspberries

1 **banana**, very cold or frozen
for 1 hour, cut in pieces

¼ cup (60 ml) grated,
unsweetened coconut

4 fresh mint leaves

METHOD

In a blender or food processor, combine all ingredients and blend for 20 to 35 seconds or until smooth.

Add water or almond milk as needed for a smoother consistency.

Nutrition Facts Per serving	
Amount	% Daily Value
Calories 230	
Fat 9 g	14%
Saturated 7 g + Trans 0 g	
Polyunsaturated 0.4 g	
Omega-6 0.3 g	
Omega-3 0.1 g	
Monounsaturated 0.4 g	
Cholesterol 1 mg	0%
Sodium 40 mg	2%
Potassium 370 mg	11%
Carbohydrates 26 g	9%
Fiber 7 g	28%
Sugar 13 g	
Protein 10 g	
Vitamin A 44 ER	4%
Vitamin C 23 mg	40%
Calcium 89 mg	8%
Iron 1.2 mg	8%
Phosphorus 59 mg	6%

RASPBERRY SPINACH
SMOOTHIE

2 SERVINGS

5 MINUTES

INGREDIENTS

¼ cup (60 ml) almond milk or water

⅔ cup (160 ml) plain Greek yogurt

1 cup (250 ml) baby **spinach**

½ cucumber, peeled, seeded and cut in pieces

1 stalk celery, in pieces

1 cup (250 ml) fresh or frozen raspberries

1 tsp chia seeds

3 to 5 ice cubes

METHOD

In a blender or food processor, combine all ingredients and blend for 20 to 35 seconds or until smooth.

Add water or almond milk as needed for a smoother consistency.

Nutrition Facts Per serving	
Amount	**% Daily Value**
Calories 110	
Fat 1 g	2%
Saturated 0.2 g + Trans 0 g	
Polyunsaturated 0.5 g	
Omega-6 0.3 g	
Omega-3 0.4 g	
Monounsaturated 0.1 g	
Cholesterol 1 mg	0%
Sodium 75 mg	3%
Potassium 250 mg	7%
Carbohydrates 13 g	4%
Fiber 6 g	24%
Sugar 7 g	
Protein 11 g	
Vitamin A 20 ER	2%
Vitamin C 20 mg	35%
Calcium 126 mg	10%
Iron 0.8 mg	6%
Phosphorus 51.3 mg	4%

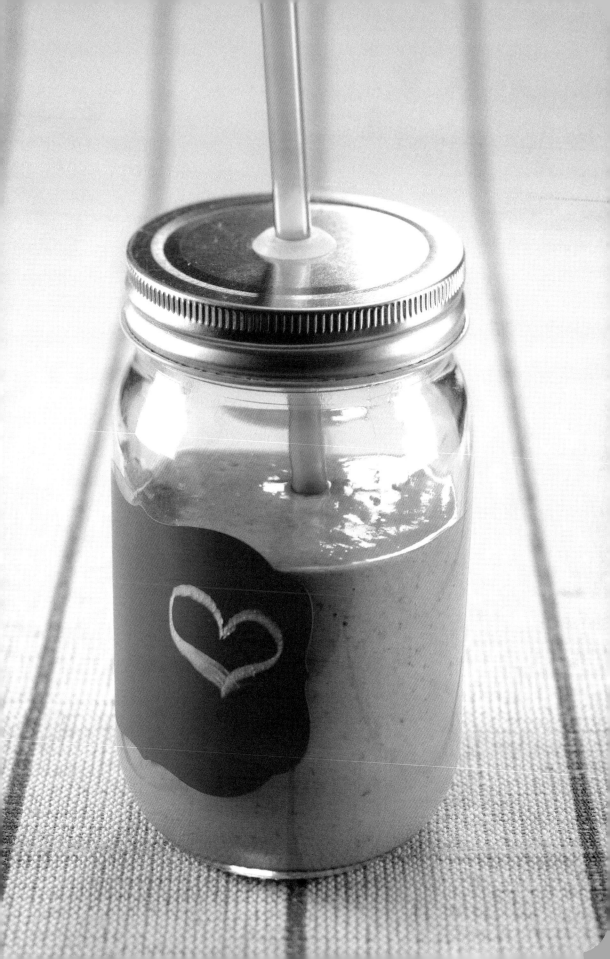

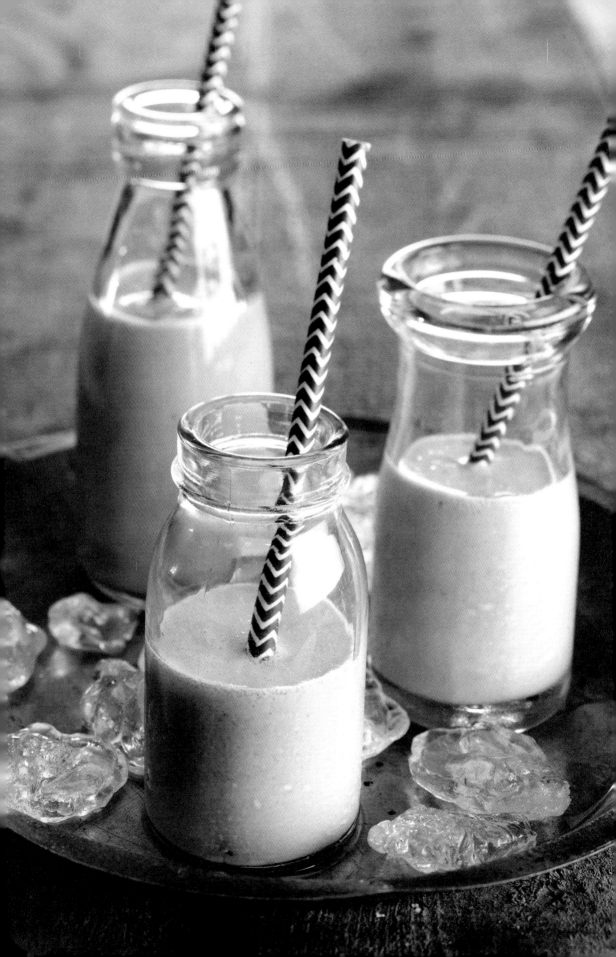

BANANA AND GREEN TEA
SMOOTHIE

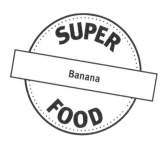

2 SERVINGS

5 MINUTES

Banana

SUPER FOOD

INGREDIENTS

1½ cups (375 ml) almond milk

½ cup (125 ml) cold green tea

½ cup (125 ml) plain Greek yogurt

1 ripe **banana,** in pieces

2 tbsp almond or peanut butter

3 to 5 ice cubes

METHOD

In a blender or food processor, combine all ingredients and blend for 20 to 35 seconds or until smooth.

Add water or almond milk as needed for a smoother consistency.

Nutrition Facts Per serving		
Amount		**% Daily Value**
Calories 210		
Fat 10 g		15%
Saturated 1 g		
+ Trans 0 g		
Polyunsaturated 2 g		
Omega-6 2 g		
Omega-3 0.1 g		
Monounsaturated 6 g		
Cholesterol 1 mg		0%
Sodium 40 mg		2%
Potassium 350 mg		10%
Carbohydrates 19 g		6%
Fiber 2 g		8%
Sugar 9 g		
Protein 10 g		
Vitamin A 4 ER		0%
Vitamin C 5 mg		8%
Calcium 107 mg		10%
Iron 0.8 mg		6%
Phosphorus 96.1 mg		8%

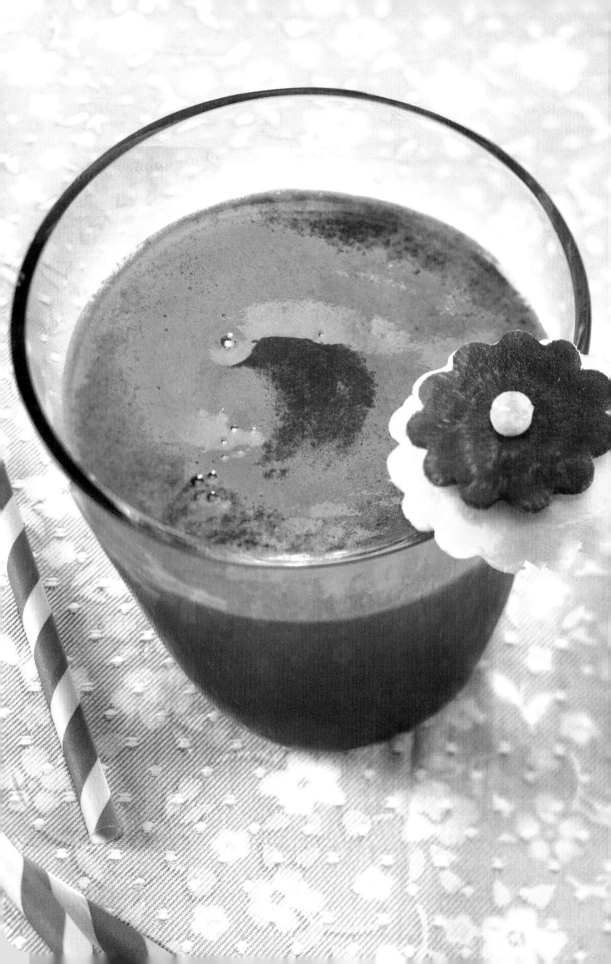

BEET AND RED GRAPE
JUICE

2 SERVINGS
5 MINUTES

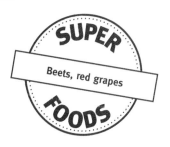

SUPER
Beets, red grapes
FOODS

INGREDIENTS

3 small **beets**,
unpeeled, washed

2 cups (500 ml) carrots,
unpeeled, washed

1 cup (250 ml) **red grapes**

1 small apple, unpeeled

Juice of 1 lemon

1 tbsp chopped fresh ginger

METHOD

In a juicer, juice beets, carrots, grapes and apple.

Add lemon juice and ginger. Mix well.

Nutrition Facts Per serving	
Amount	**% Daily Value**
Calories 190	
Fat 0.5 g	1%
Saturated 0.1 g	
+ Trans 0 g	
Polyunsaturated 0.3 g	
Omega-6 0.3 g	
Omega-3 0 g	
Monounsaturated 0.1 g	
Cholesterol 0 mg	0%
Sodium 190 mg	8%
Potassium 1030 mg	29%
Carbohydrates 43 g	14%
Fiber 2 g	8%
Sugar 28 g	
Protein 4 g	
Vitamin A 787 ER	80%
Vitamin C 41 mg	70%
Calcium 74 mg	6%
Iron 1.7 mg	10%
Phosphorus 114.2 mg	10%

——— DID YOU KNOW? ———

Beets get their color from betalains. These pigments are eliminated in urine and stools, which can take on a reddish color.

79

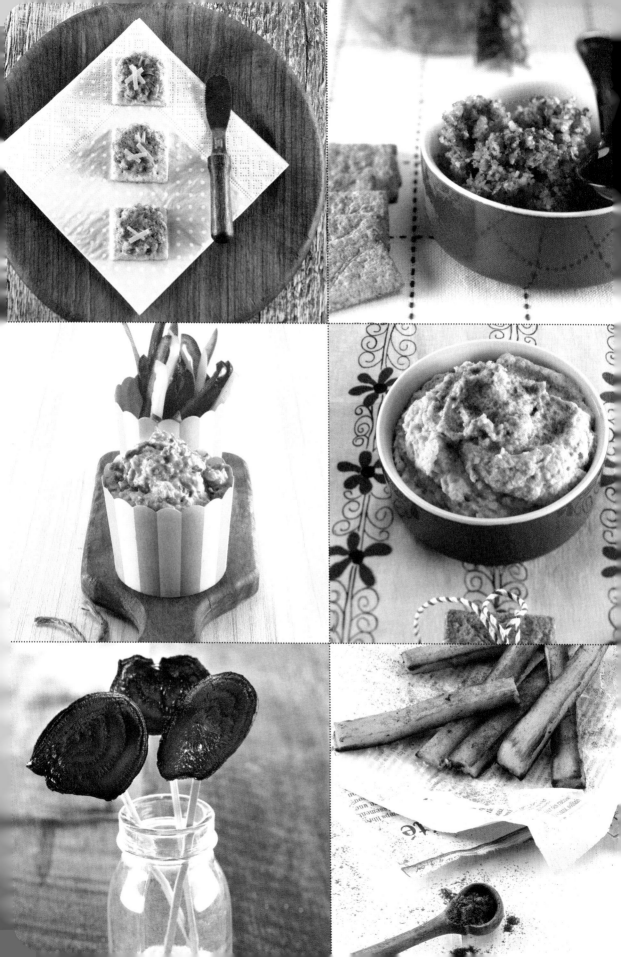

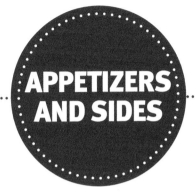

APPETIZERS AND SIDES

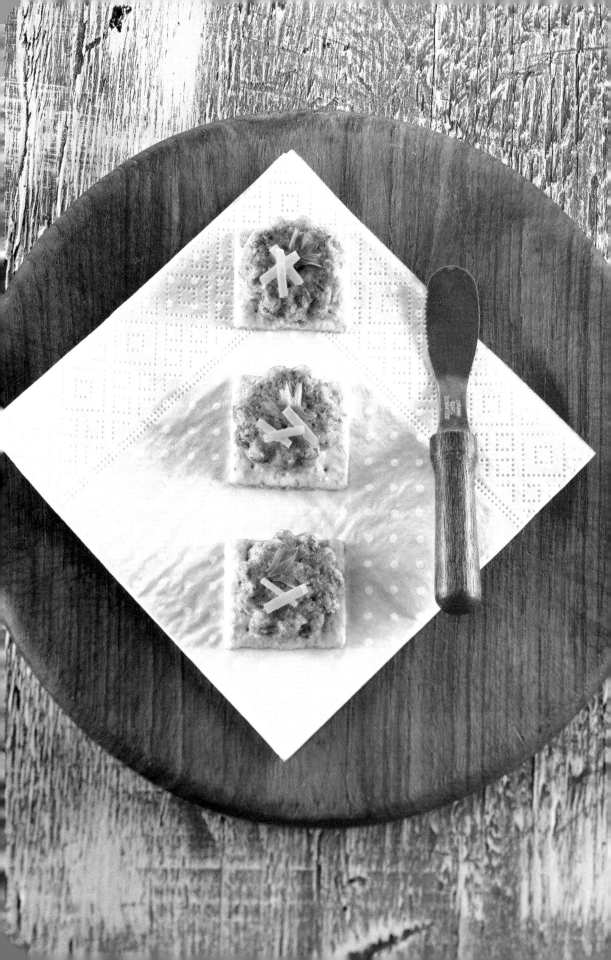

RAW VEGETARIAN
BREAKFAST SPREAD

16 SERVINGS
10 MINUTES
2 HOURS

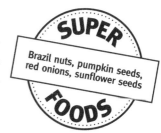

Brazil nuts, pumpkin seeds, red onions, sunflower seeds

INGREDIENTS

2 tbsp olive oil

Juice of ½ lemon

1 cup (250 ml) **sunflower seeds**

¼ cup (60 ml) **Brazil nuts**

¼ cup (60 ml) **pumpkin seeds**

¼ cup (60 ml) grated carrots

¼ **red onion,** chopped

1 clove garlic, finely chopped

1 tbsp yeast (optional)

1 tbsp grated fresh ginger

1 tbsp chopped fresh oregano

1 tbsp chopped fresh parsley

Seasoning to taste

METHOD

In a food processor, process ingredients until they form a ball. If mixture is too dry, add a bit more lemon juice. Adjust seasoning.

Pour mixture into a 9 x 9 inch (23 x 23 cm) mold and refrigerate for about 2 hours.

Cut into 16 portions.

Serve with whole-grain crackers.

Nutrition Facts Per serving	
Amount	% Daily Value
Calories 80	
Fat 7 g	11%
Saturated 1 g	
+ Trans 0 g	
Polyunsaturated 3.5 g	
Omega-6 3.5 g	
Omega-3 0 g	
Monounsaturated 2 g	
Cholesterol 0 mg	0%
Sodium 2 mg	0%
Potassium 70 mg	2%
Carbohydrates 3 g	1%
Fiber 1 g	4%
Sugar 1 g	
Protein 2 g	
Vitamin A 25 ER	2%
Vitamin C 2 mg	4%
Calcium 12 mg	2%
Iron 0.8 mg	6%
Phosphorus 105.7 mg	10%

BEET
CHIPS

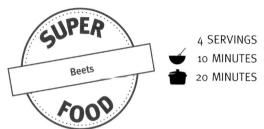

SUPER
Beets
FOOD

- 4 SERVINGS
- 10 MINUTES
- 20 MINUTES

INGREDIENTS

4 **beets**, very thinly sliced

2 tbsp olive oil

4 sprigs rosemary, chopped

Seasoning to taste

METHOD

Position rack in center of oven and preheat to 350°F (180°C). Line a baking sheet with parchment paper.

In a bowl, combine all ingredients.

Lay sliced beets on prepared baking sheet. Bake in center of preheated oven for 15 to 20 minutes or until crispy.

Let cool on baking sheet.

--- **DID YOU KNOW?** ---

Red beets are used as coloring in the food industry. There are also yellow beets and white beets with red veining. White beets are mainly used to make sugar. They are called the "sugar beet."

Nutrition Facts Per serving

Amount	% Daily Value
Calories 90	
Fat 7 g	11%
Saturated 1 g	
+ Trans 0 g	
Polyunsaturated 0.5 g	
Omega-6 0.5 g	
Omega-3 0.1 g	
Monounsaturated 5 g	
Cholesterol 0 mg	0%
Sodium 40 mg	2%
Potassium 150 mg	4%
Carbohydrates 5 g	2%
Fiber 1 g	4%
Sugar 4 g	
Protein 1 g	
Vitamin A 2 ER	0%
Vitamin C 2 mg	4%
Calcium 8 mg	0%
Iron 0.4 mg	4%
Phosphorus 19 mg	2%

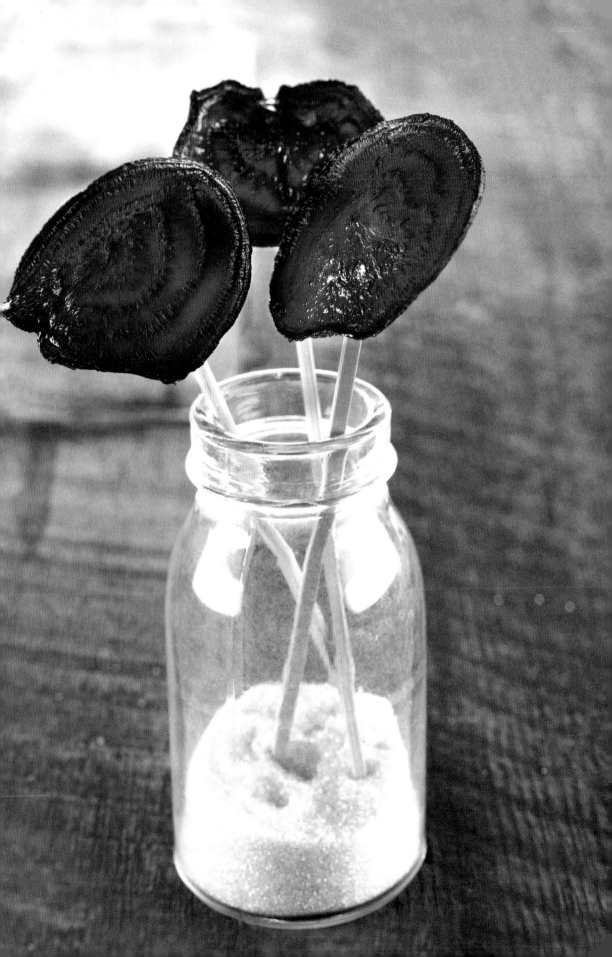

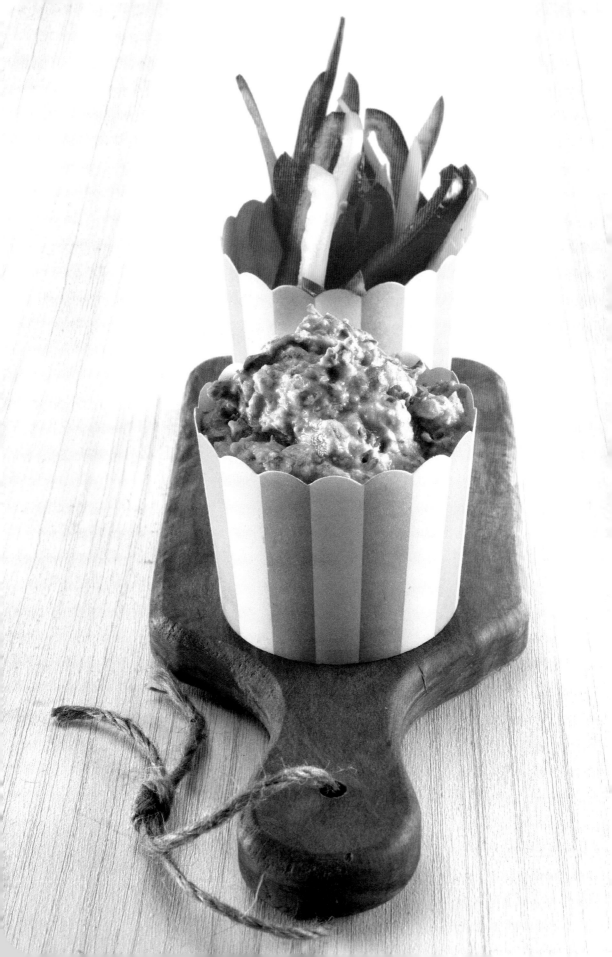

PUMPKIN SEED
GUACAMOLE

8 SERVINGS OF ¼ cup (60 ml)

🥣 15 MINUTES

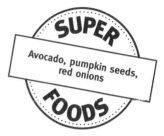

SUPER FOODS

Avocado, pumpkin seeds, red onions

INGREDIENTS

2 very ripe **avocados**

Juice of 1 lime

1 tomato, finely chopped

1 small **red onion**, finely chopped

¼ cup (60 ml) **pumpkin seeds**, ground

½ cup (125 ml) fresh parsley, chopped

¼ tsp ground cumin

A few drops Tabasco sauce

Seasoning to taste

METHOD

In a blender, purée avocado flesh with lime juice for about 2 minutes.

In a bowl, combine avocado purée and remaining ingredients. Refrigerate until ready to serve.

Serve with whole-grain crackers or raw veggies.

COMMON MISCONCEPTIONS
Avocado is a source of bad fat.
FALSE. Avocado is one of the highest calorie and highest fat fruits, but a large part of the fat is monounsaturated: a great health ally.

Nutrition Facts
Per serving

Amount	% Daily Value
Calories 140	
Fat 10 g	15%
Saturated 2 g	
+ Trans 0 g	
Polyunsaturated 2 g	
Omega-6 2 g	
Omega-3 0.1 g	
Monounsaturated 5 g	
Cholesterol 0 mg	0%
Sodium 10 mg	0%
Potassium 380 mg	11%
Carbohydrates 9 g	3%
Fiber 5 g	20%
Sugar 3 g	
Protein 4 g	
Vitamin A 58 ER	6%
Vitamin C 24 mg	40%
Calcium 20 mg	2%
Iron 1.2 mg	8%
Phosphorus 91.7 mg	8%

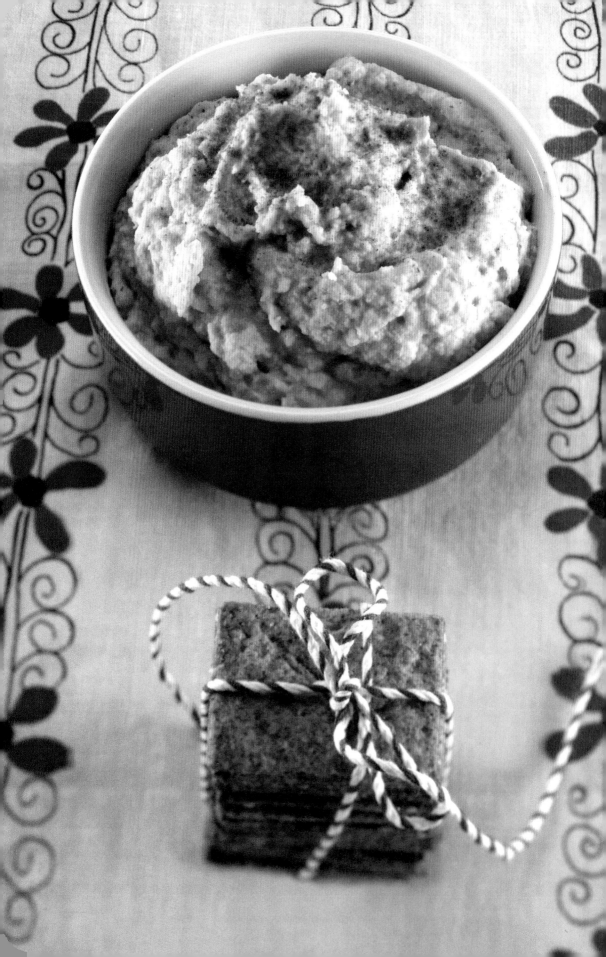

SUNFLOWER SEED
HUMMUS

15 SERVINGS OF ¼ cup (60 ml)

🥣 10 MINUTES

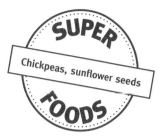

SUPER FOODS

Chickpeas, sunflower seeds

INGREDIENTS

½ cup (125 ml) freshly squeezed lemon juice

1 can (19 oz/540 ml) **chickpeas**, drained and rinsed

¼ cup (60 ml) tahini (sesame butter)

¼ cup (60 ml) **sunflower seeds**

2 cloves garlic, finely chopped

1 tbsp chopped fresh basil

1 tsp ground cumin

Drizzle olive oil

Pinch paprika

Seasoning to taste

METHOD

In a food processor, process all ingredients, except oil and paprika, for 1 minute or until smooth. Adjust seasoning.

Before serving, add a drizzle of oil and stir. Sprinkle with paprika.

Serve with whole-grain crackers or raw veggies.

Nutrition Facts Per serving	
Amount	**% Daily Value**
Calories 90	
Fat 5 g	8%
Saturated 0.5 g + Trans 0 g	
Polyunsaturated 2 g	
Omega-6 2 g	
Omega-3 0 g	
Monounsaturated 2 g	
Cholesterol 0 mg	0%
Sodium 5 mg	0%
Potassium 115 mg	13%
Carbohydrates 9 g	3%
Fiber 2 g	8%
Sugar 1 g	
Protein 3 g	
Vitamin A 3 ER	0%
Vitamin C 4 mg	8%
Calcium 33 mg	4%
Iron 1.1 mg	8%
Phosphorus 101.1 mg	10%

SPINACH AND WALNUT
PESTO

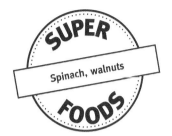

20 SERVINGS OF 1 tbsp

 10 MINUTES

 12 MINUTES

INGREDIENTS

2 cups (500 ml) **walnuts**

3 cups (750 ml) roughly torn **spinach**

1 cup (250 ml) fresh basil

2 tbsp grated Parmesan

½ cup (125 ml) olive oil

Seasoning to taste

METHOD

Preheat oven to 350°F (180°C).

Spread nuts on a baking sheet and roast in preheated oven for 12 minutes or until golden.

In a food processor, process nuts and remaining ingredients, except oil and seasonings, for 1 minute or until blended.

Add oil in a stream while mixing, until desired consistency is reached. Season.

Serve with whole-grain crackers or raw veggies.

SPINACH: FRESH, FROZEN OR CANNED?

Fresh and frozen spinach are the best choices. Canned spinach is generally overcooked and has a slightly metallic taste.

Nutrition Facts Per serving	
Amount	% Daily Value
Calories 130	
Fat 13 g	20%
Saturated 1.5 g	
+ Trans 0 g	
Polyunsaturated 6 g	
Omega-6 5 g	
Omega-3 1 g	
Monounsaturated 5 g	
Cholesterol 1 mg	0%
Sodium 10 mg	0%
Potassium 70 mg	2%
Carbohydrates 2 g	1%
Fiber 1 g	4%
Sugar 0 g	
Protein 2 g	
Vitamin A 26 ER	2%
Vitamin C 1 mg	2%
Calcium 23 mg	2%
Iron 0.5 mg	4%
Phosphorus 48.3 mg	4%

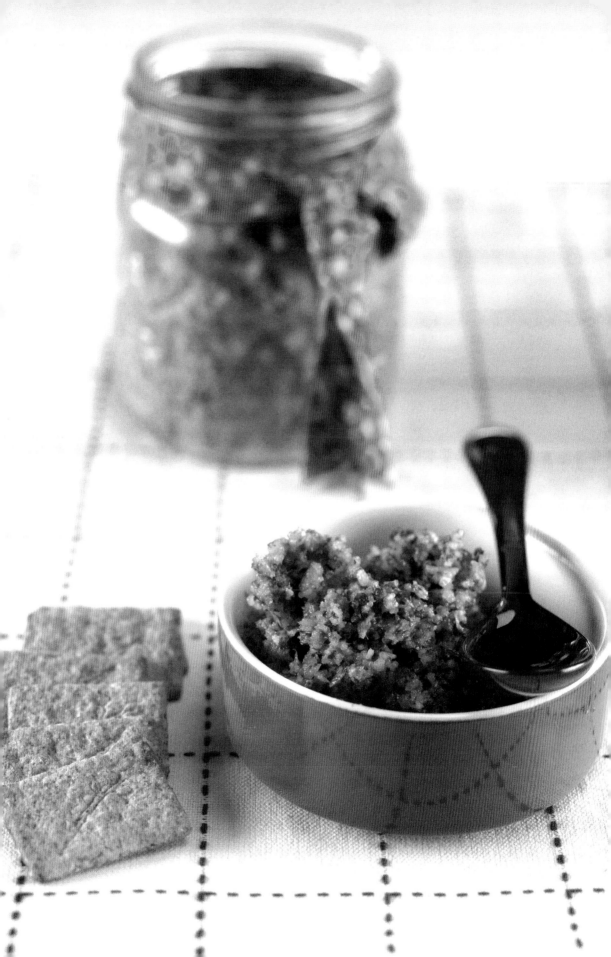

BEET AND KALE
QUINOA

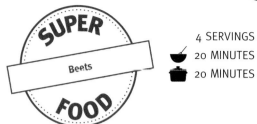

SUPER
Beets
FOOD

4 SERVINGS
20 MINUTES
20 MINUTES

INGREDIENTS

2 cups (500 ml) water

1 cup (250 ml) quinoa, rinsed and drained

2 tbsp olive oil

2 cloves garlic, finely chopped

4 **beets**, peeled and diced

2 tsp cumin seeds, lightly crushed

4 kale leaves, without stem, torn

¼ cup (60 ml) chopped fresh cilantro

½ cup (125 ml) crumbled goat cheese

Seasoning to taste

METHOD

In a large saucepan over medium heat, bring water to a boil and add quinoa. Reduce heat to low. Cover and simmer for 12 minutes. Drain.

Meanwhile, heat oil in a large, heavy-bottomed pan over medium heat and sauté garlic and beets for 3 to 5 minutes. Add cumin, kale and cilantro. Stir for 30 to 60 seconds.

Add quinoa and gently combine until distributed throughout. Season.

Pour mixture in a bowl or a large plate. Top with goat cheese. Serve hot or cold.

Nutrition Facts Per serving	
Amount	**% Daily Value**
Calories 390	
Fat 17 g	26%
Saturated 6 g	
+ Trans 0 g	
Polyunsaturated 2 g	
Omega-6 2 g	
Omega-3 0.2 g	
Monounsaturated 7 g	
Cholesterol 20 mg	7%
Sodium 140 mg	6%
Potassium 850 mg	24%
Carbohydrates 43 g	14%
Fiber 6 g	24%
Sugar 7 g	
Protein 15 g	
Vitamin A 668 ER	70%
Vitamin C 33 mg	55%
Calcium 321 mg	30%
Iron 7.9 mg	60%
Phosphorus 394.5 mg	35%

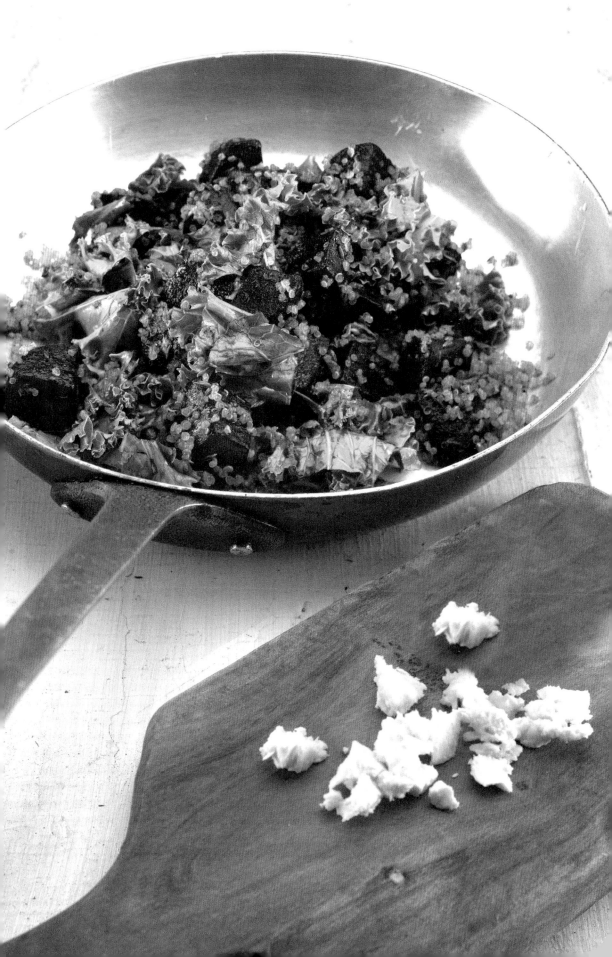

BAKED SWEET POTATO
FRIES

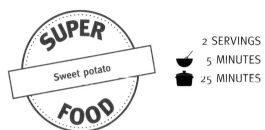

SUPER
Sweet potato
FOOD

2 SERVINGS
5 MINUTES
25 MINUTES

INGREDIENTS

2 medium **sweet potatoes,**
in strips

2 tbsp olive oil

1 tbsp paprika

Seasoning to taste

METHOD

Position rack in center of oven and preheat to 400°F (200°C).

In a large bowl, combine all ingredients.

Place sweet potatoes on an oiled baking sheet. Bake in center of preheated oven, turning partway through cooking, for about 20 minutes.

Continue baking for 3 to 5 minutes or until fries are crispy.

Nutrition Facts Per serving		
Amount		**% Daily Value**
Calories 240		
Fat 13 g		20%
Saturated 2 g		
+ Trans 0 g		
Polyunsaturated 1.5 g		
Omega-6 1.5 g		
Omega-3 0.1 g		
Monounsaturated 10 g		
Cholesterol 0 mg		0%
Sodium 75 mg		3%
Potassium 510 mg		15%
Carbohydrates 28 g		9%
Fiber 5 g		20%
Sugar 6 g		
Protein 3 g		
Vitamin A 1007 ER		100%
Vitamin C 5 mg		10%
Calcium 45 mg		4%
Iron 1.6 mg		10%
Phosphorus 72.2 mg		6%

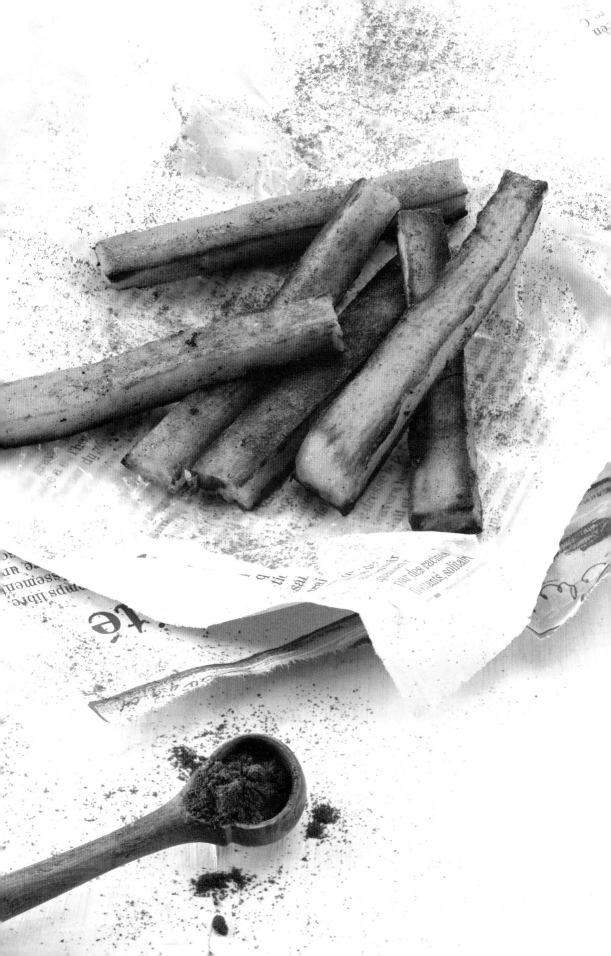

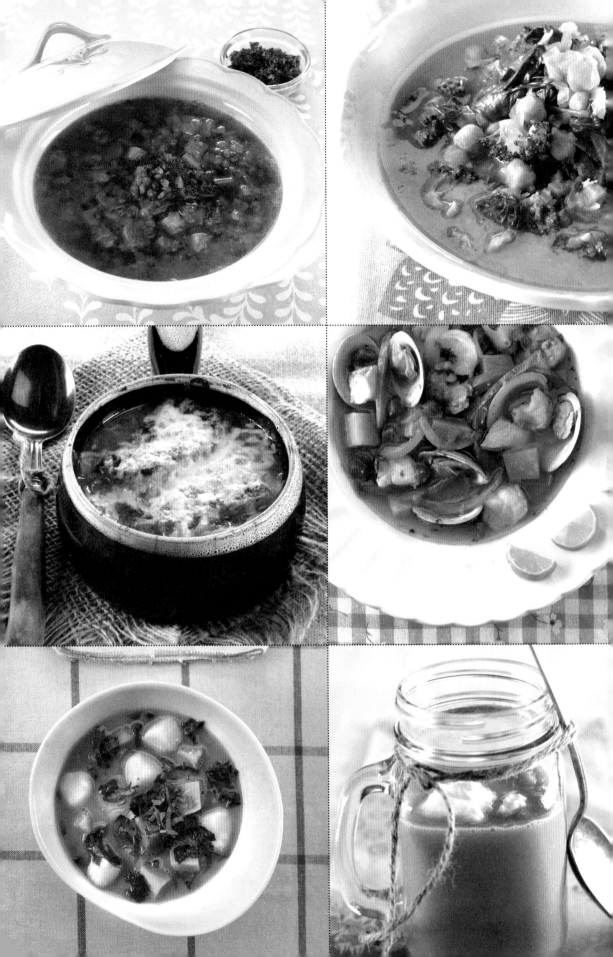

SOUPS

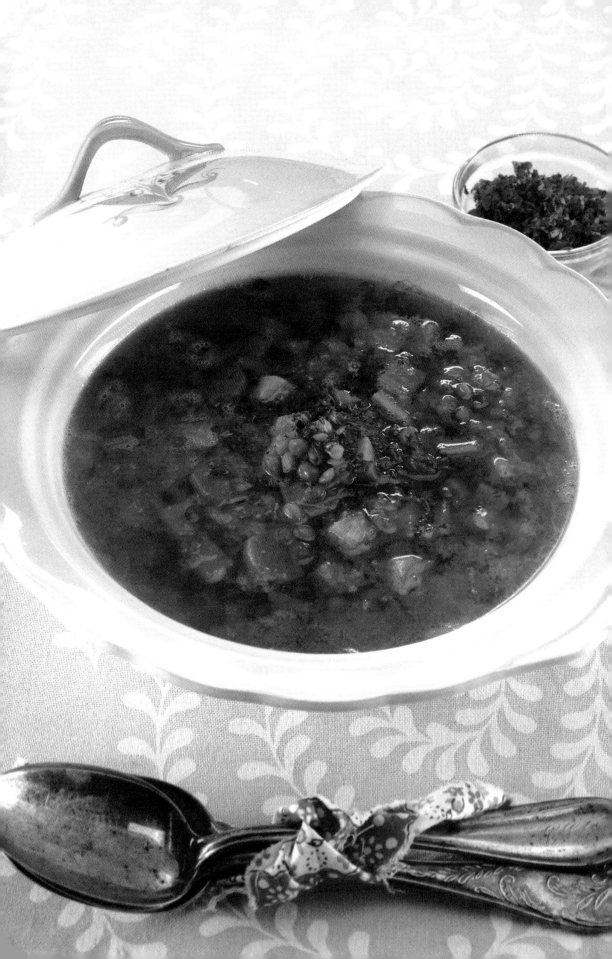

LENTIL AND SWEET POTATO
SOUP

4 SERVINGS
20 MINUTES
20 MINUTES

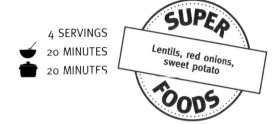

Lentils, red onions, sweet potato

INGREDIENTS

1 tbsp olive oil

2 **red onions**, finely chopped

3 cloves garlic, finely chopped

2 carrots, in rounds

1 **sweet potato**, peeled and cubed

6 cups (1.5 liters) chicken or vegetable broth

1 can (19 oz/540 ml) **lentils**, drained and rinsed

½ tsp curry powder

2 tbsp chopped fresh parsley

Seasoning to taste

METHOD

In a large saucepan, heat oil over medium heat and sauté onions, garlic, carrots and sweet potato for 3 to 5 minutes.

Add broth, lentils and curry. Reduce heat to low. Cover and simmer for 12 to 15 minutes.

Add parsley and season.

Nutrition Facts Per serving	
Amount	**% Daily Value**
Calories 230	
Fat 4 g	6%
Saturated 0.5 g + Trans 0 g	
Polyunsaturated 0.5 g	
Omega-6 0.5 g	
Omega-3 0.1 g	
Monounsaturated 2.5 g	
Cholesterol 0 mg	0%
Sodium 150 mg	6%
Potassium 910 mg	26%
Carbohydrates 37 g	12%
Fiber 6 g	24%
Sugar 10 g	
Protein 11 g	
Vitamin A 963 ER	100%
Vitamin C 12 mg	20%
Calcium 62 mg	6%
Iron 3.3 mg	25%
Phosphorus 194.6 mg	20%

DID YOU KNOW?
Legumes can help you lose weight. They are nourishing, filling and high in protein and fiber, but low in fat.

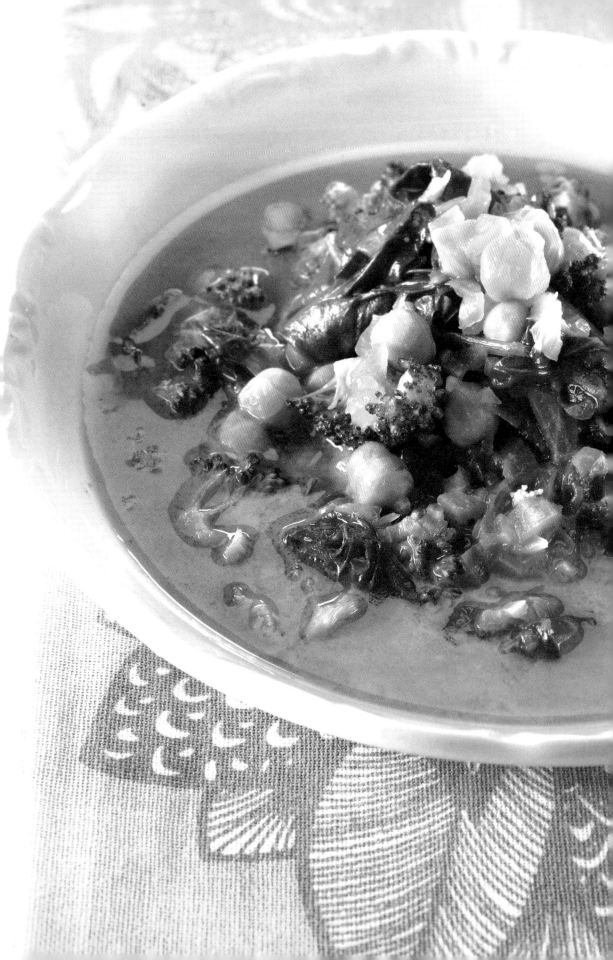

CHICKPEA, SPINACH
AND BROCCOLI SOUP

4 SERVINGS
15 MINUTES
20 MINUTES

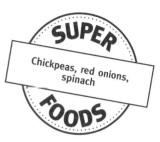

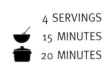
Chickpeas, red onions, spinach

INGREDIENTS

1 tbsp olive oil

2 **red onions**, finely chopped

2 cloves garlic, finely chopped

4 cups (1 liter) baby **spinach**

2 cups (500 ml) broccoli florets

3 sprigs fresh thyme

3 cups (750 ml) chicken or vegetable broth

1 can (14 oz/398 ml) coconut milk

1 can (19 oz/540 ml) **chickpeas**, drained and rinsed

1 tsp ground turmeric

Seasoning to taste

METHOD

In a large saucepan, heat oil over medium heat and sauté onions and garlic for 3 to 5 minutes.

Add spinach, broccoli, thyme, broth and coconut milk. Continue cooking for 10 minutes.

Add chickpeas and turmeric. Continue cooking for 5 minutes and season.

Nutrition Facts Per serving	
Amount	**% Daily Value**
Calories 270	
Fat 6 g	9%
Saturated 1 g + Trans 0 g	
Polyunsaturated 1.5 g	
Omega-6 1.5 g	
Omega-3 0.1 g	
Monounsaturated 3 g	
Cholesterol 0 mg	0%
Sodium 200 mg	8%
Potassium 1050 mg	30%
Carbohydrates 40 g	13%
Fiber 8 g	32%
Sugar 11 g	
Protein 13 g	
Vitamin A 328 ER	35%
Vitamin C 30 mg	50%
Calcium 145 mg	15%
Iron 5 mg	35%
Phosphorus 239.2 mg	20%

ONION SOUP
AU GRATIN

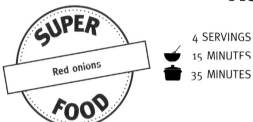

SUPER
Red onions
FOOD

🥣 4 SERVINGS
15 MINUTES
🍲 35 MINUTES

INGREDIENTS

2 tbsp olive oil

4 **red onions,** finely chopped

3 cups (750 ml) chicken or vegetable broth

1 cup (250 ml) water

1 bay leaf

4 slices toast (optional)

1 cup (250 ml) grated cheese

Seasoning to taste

METHOD

In a saucepan, heat oil over medium heat and sauté onions, stirring occasionally, for 10 minutes or until golden.

Add broth, water and bay leaf and bring to a boil. Reduce heat to low. Cover and simmer for 20 minutes or until onions are tender. Season.

Divide soup into 4 ovenproof bowls. Cover with toast, if using, and top with cheese. Place under preheated oven broiler for a few minutes until cheese is melted and browned.

Nutrition Facts Per serving	
Amount	**% Daily Value**
Calories 290	
Fat 13 g	20%
Saturated 4.5 g	
+ Trans 0.2 g	
Polyunsaturated 1 g	
Omega-6 1 g	
Omega-3 0.1 g	
Monounsaturated 7 g	
Cholesterol 15 mg	5%
Sodium 350 mg	14%
Potassium 440 mg	13%
Carbohydrates 30 g	10%
Fiber 4 g	16%
Sugar 14 g	
Protein 13 g	
Vitamin A 41 ER	4%
Vitamin C 10 mg	15%
Calcium 249 mg	25%
Iron 1.4 mg	10%
Phosphorus 248.9 mg	25%

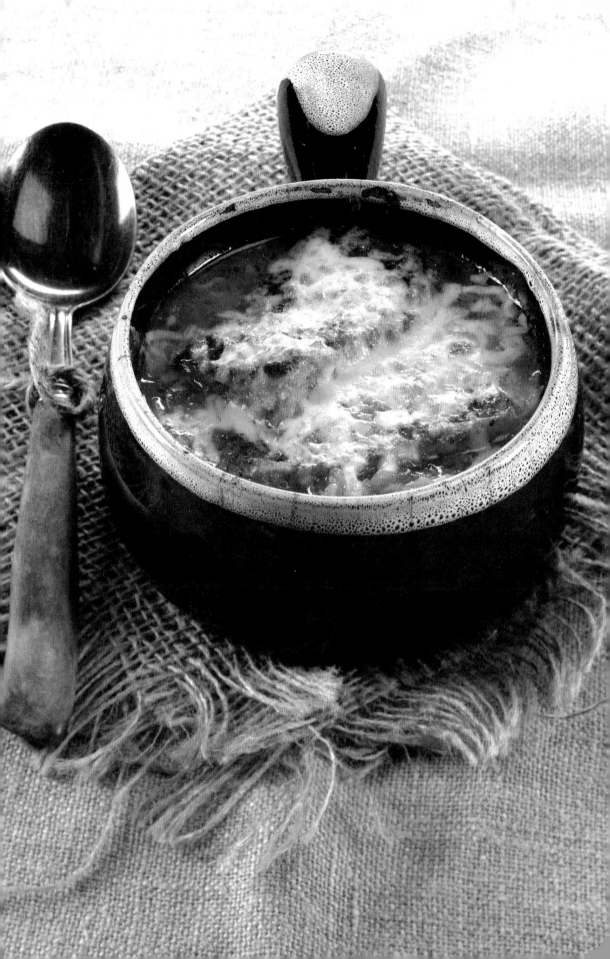

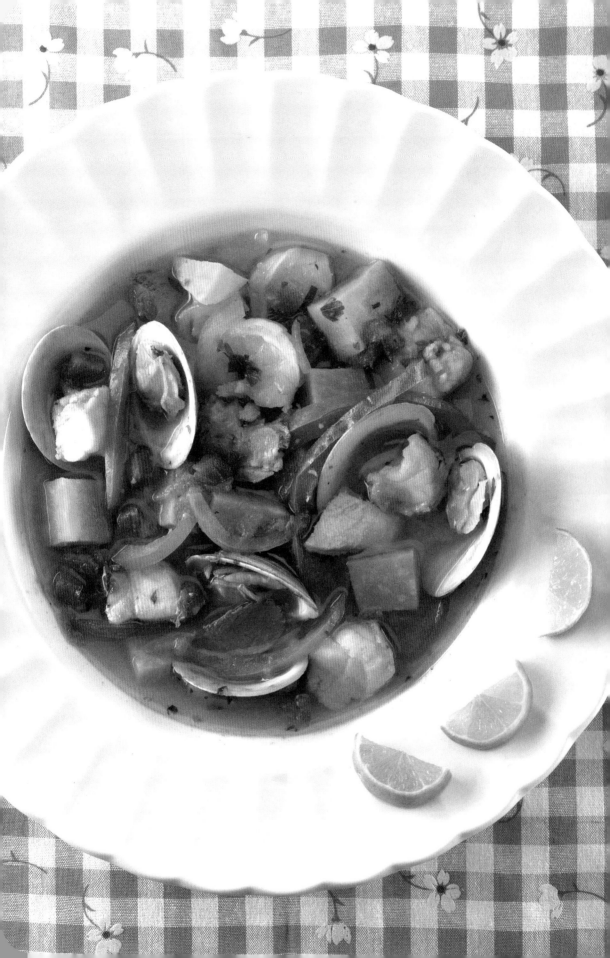

MEDITERRANEAN FISH
AND VEGETABLE SOUP

6 SERVINGS
20 MINUTES
2 HOURS
30 MINUTES

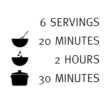

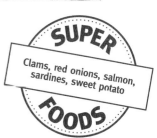

Clams, red onions, salmon, sardines, sweet potato

INGREDIENTS

20 hard-shell **clams**

1 **red onion**, finely chopped

4 cloves garlic, finely chopped

1 red pepper, in strips

1 green pepper, in strips

2 cups (500 ml) diced ripe tomatoes

½ cup (125 ml) chopped fresh parsley

2 bay leaves

4 **sweet potatoes**, peeled and cubed

20 raw shrimp, peeled

10 oz (300 g) fresh **salmon**, cubed

10 oz (300 g) monkfish (or other white fish), in large cubes

2 tbsp tomato paste

1 cup (250 ml) white wine

1 cup (250 ml) vegetable or fish broth

5 cups (1.25 liters) water

2 tbsp olive oil

½ tsp crushed red pepper flakes

2 cans (each 3.5 oz/100 g) **sardines** in water (optional)

Handful fresh mint leaves, torn

Seasoning to taste

METHOD

Wash clams. Soak in a large bowl of cold water for 2 hours, changing water two or three times. Rinse well and drain. (Do not transfer contents of bowl to a strainer; otherwise sand settled at bottom will be poured over clams).

In a large saucepan, combine clams, onion, garlic, peppers, tomatoes, parsley and bay leaves. Cover with sweet potatoes, shrimp, salmon and monkfish.

Add tomato paste, wine, broth, water, oil and chiles. Season and combine. Cover and simmer over low heat for 25 minutes.

Add sardines, if using, and mint. Continue cooking for about 5 minutes. Remove bay leaves.

Nutrition Facts Per serving		
Amount		**% Daily Value**
Calories 410		
Fat 15 g		23%
Saturated 2.5 g		
+ Trans 0 g		
Polyunsaturated 4.5 g		
Omega-6 2.5 g		
Omega-3 2 g		
Monounsaturated 7 g		
Cholesterol 160 mg		53%
Sodium 500 mg		21%
Potassium 1300 mg		37%
Carbohydrates 27 g		9%
Fiber 4 g		16%
Sugar 7 g		
Protein 41 g		
Vitamin A 721 ER		70%
Vitamin C 30 mg		50%
Calcium 249 mg		25%
Iron 1.1 mg		8%
Phosphorus 581.7 mg		50%

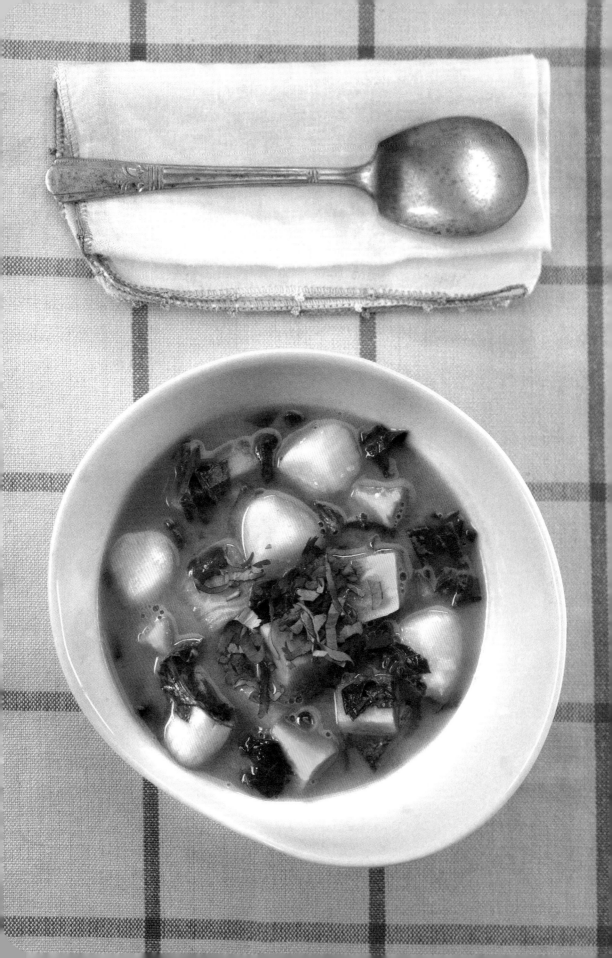

SCALLOP, SWEET POTATO
AND SPINACH SOUP

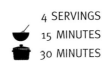

4 SERVINGS
15 MINUTES
30 MINUTES

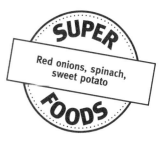

Red onions, spinach, sweet potato

INGREDIENTS

1 tbsp olive oil

1 **red onion**, finely chopped

8 cloves garlic, finely chopped

1 **sweet potato**, peeled and cubed

6 cups (1.5 liters) chicken or vegetable broth

Juice of 1 lime or 1 lemon

1 lb (454 g) scallops

4 cups (1 liter) coarsely chopped **spinach**

2 tbsp chopped fresh cilantro

Seasoning to taste

METHOD

In a large saucepan, heat oil over high heat and sauté onion, garlic and sweet potato for 5 minutes.

Add broth and lime juice. Reduce heat to medium. Cover and cook for 20 minutes.

Add scallops and spinach. Continue cooking for about 5 minutes and season.

When ready to serve, garnish with cilantro. Season.

Nutrition Facts Per serving	
Amount	**% Daily Value**
Calories 220	
Fat 4.5 g	7%
Saturated 0.5 g + Trans 0 g	
Polyunsaturated 0.5 g	
Omega-6 0.4 g	
Omega-3 0.3 g	
Monounsaturated 2.5 g	
Cholesterol 35 mg	12%
Sodium 330 mg	14%
Potassium 1040 mg	30%
Carbohydrates 21 g	7%
Fiber 2 g	8%
Sugar 6 g	
Protein 24 g	
Vitamin A 727 ER	40%
Vitamin C 32 mg	50%
Calcium 99 mg	8%
Iron 1.9 mg	15%
Phosphorus 303.5 mg	30%

CLAM
CHOWARD

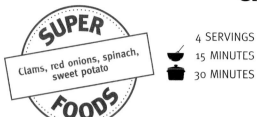

SUPER FOODS

Clams, red onions, spinach, sweet potato

4 SERVINGS
15 MINUTES
30 MINUTES

INGREDIENTS

3 **sweet potatoes**, peeled and chopped in 1-inch (2.5 cm) dice

1 tbsp olive oil

1 **red onion**, diced

4 cloves garlic, finely chopped

1 stalk celery, diced

1 yellow pepper, diced

1 leek, in thin rounds

2 cups (500 ml) vegetable or fish broth

1 cup (250 ml) milk or unsweetened soy or almond milk

½ cup (125 ml) white wine

Juice of 1 lemon

1 large tomato, chopped

2 tbsp fresh thyme

¼ tsp cayenne pepper

¼ tsp paprika

2 tbsp chopped fresh dill

¼ cup (60 ml) chopped fresh cilantro

1 cup (250 ml) baby **spinach**

2 lbs (1 kg) **clams**, properly cleaned

Seasoning to taste

METHOD

Wash clams. Soak in a large bowl of cold water for 2 hours, changing water two or three times. Rinse well and drain. (Do not transfer contents of bowl to a strainer; otherwise sand settled at bottom will be poured over clams).

In a steamer basket over medium heat, cook sweet potatoes, covered, for 15 to 20 minutes.

Meanwhile, in another saucepan, heat oil over medium heat and sauté onion, garlic, celery, pepper and leek for 7 minutes.

Add broth, milk, wine, lemon juice, tomato, thyme, cayenne pepper, paprika, dill, cilantro and cooked sweet potatoes. Adjust seasoning and bring to a boil.

Add spinach and clams. Cook over medium heat for a few minutes. Chowder is ready once clams open.

Nutrition Facts Per serving	
Amount	% Daily Value
Calories 310	
Fat 6 g	9%
Saturated 1 g	
+ Trans 0 g	
Polyunsaturated 1.5 g	
Omega-6 1 g	
Omega-3 0.2 g	
Monounsaturated 3 g	
Cholesterol 10 mg	3%
Sodium 260 mg	11%
Potassium 1450 mg	41%
Carbohydrates 50 g	17%
Fiber 9 g	36%
Sugar 14 g	
Protein 13 g	
Vitamin A 797 ER	80%
Vitamin C 47 mg	80%
Calcium 298 mg	25%
Iron 5.5 mg	40%
Phosphorus 251.3 mg	25%

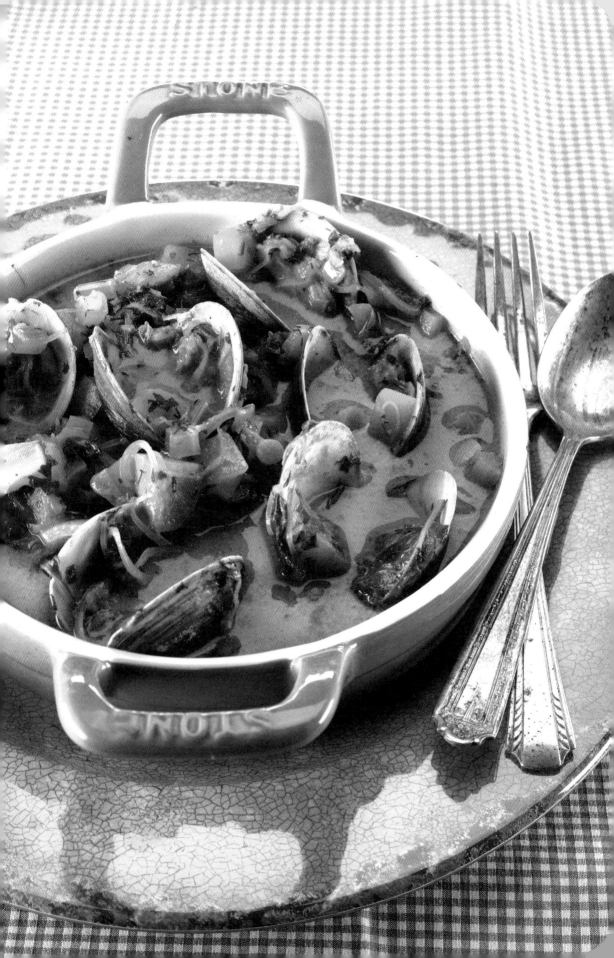

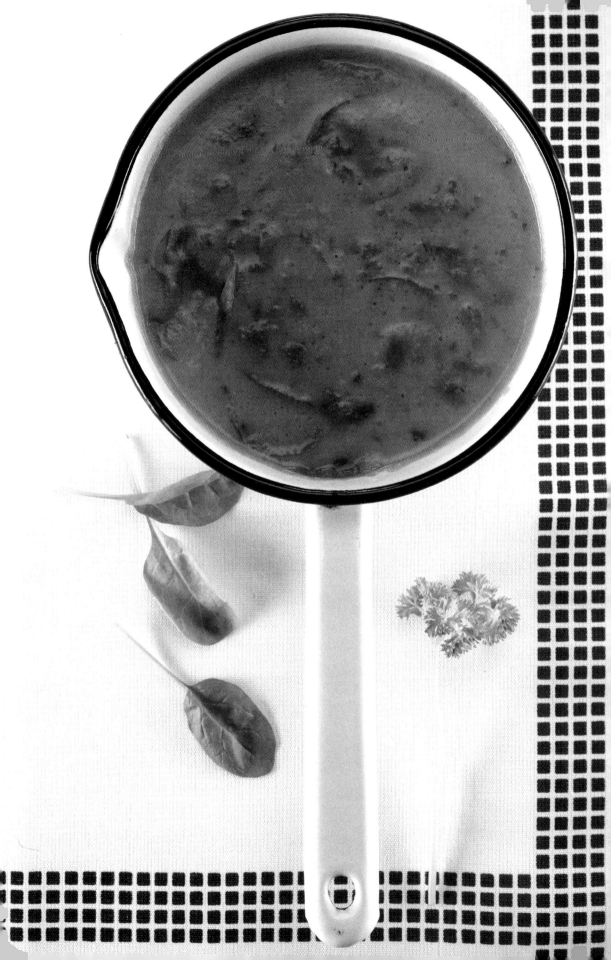

CREAM OF SPINACH
AND PINTO BEAN SOUP

4 SERVINGS
15 MINUTES
40 MINUTES

Pinto beans, red onions, spinach

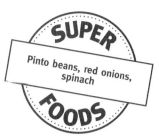

INGREDIENTS

1 tbsp olive oil

1 large **red onion**, finely chopped

2 cloves garlic, finely chopped

3 carrots, sliced in rounds

2 cups (500 ml) chicken or vegetable broth

1 can (19 oz/540 ml) **pinto beans**, drained and rinsed

2 cups (500 ml) plain almond milk

2 cups (500 ml) chopped baby **spinach**

2 tbsp chopped fresh parsley

Seasoning to taste

METHOD

In a large saucepan, heat oil over medium heat and sauté onion, garlic and carrots for 3 to 5 minutes.

Add broth and bring to a boil. Reduce heat to low and continue cooking 20 to 30 minutes or until vegetables are tender.

Add beans and almond milk.

In a blender, blend mixture until smooth. Add liquid as needed.

Return mixture to saucepan and add spinach and parsley. Continue cooking, stirring occasionally, for 3 to 4 minutes. Season.

Nutrition Facts Per serving	
Amount	% Daily Value
Calories 160	
Fat 4 g	6%
Saturated 0.5 g	
+ Trans 0 g	
Polyunsaturated 0.5 g	
Omega-6 0.5 g	
Omega-3 0.2 g	
Monounsaturated 2.5 g	
Cholesterol 0 mg	0%
Sodium 350 mg	14%
Potassium 640 mg	18%
Carbohydrates 25 g	8%
Fiber 6 g	24%
Sugar 5 g	
Protein 7 g	
Vitamin A 883 ER	90%
Vitamin C 14 mg	25%
Calcium 86 mg	8%
Iron 2.1 mg	15%
Phosphorus 122.5 mg	10%

SQUASH AND SWEET POTATO
SOUP

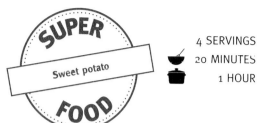

4 SERVINGS
20 MINUTES
1 HOUR

INGREDIENTS

1 medium spaghetti squash

Drizzle olive oil

4 cups (1 liter) chicken
or vegetable broth

1 medium **sweet potato**,
peeled and chopped in cubes

1 tsp roughly chopped
fresh ginger

1 tsp curry powder

1 tsp ground turmeric

4 tbsp sour cream

Seasoning to taste

METHOD

Position rack in center of oven and preheat to 350°F (180°C).

Cut squash in half lengthwise and remove seeds. On a baking sheet, place squash halves flesh-side up. Brush with oil and bake in center of preheated oven for 40 minutes or until tender. Let cool, then separate squash into strands using a fork.

Meanwhile, in a large saucepan, heat broth over medium heat. Add sweet potato and cook for 20 to 25 minutes.

Add ginger, curry, turmeric and spaghetti squash. Simmer over medium heat for 15 minutes.

In a blender, blend mixture until smooth and season.

Serve in bowls topped with sour cream.

Nutrition Facts Per serving	
Amount	% Daily Value
Calories 180	
Fat 6 g	9%
Saturated 2 g	
+ Trans 0 g	
Polyunsaturated 0.5 g	
Omega-6 0.4 g	
Omega-3 0.1 g	
Monounsaturated 2.5 g	
Cholesterol 10 mg	3%
Sodium 320 mg	13%
Potassium 950 mg	27%
Carbohydrates 23 g	8%
Fiber 3 g	12%
Sugar 12 g	
Protein 9 g	
Vitamin A 508 ER	50%
Vitamin C 5 mg	8%
Calcium 62 mg	6%
Iron 1 mg	8%
Phosphorus 36.2 mg	4%

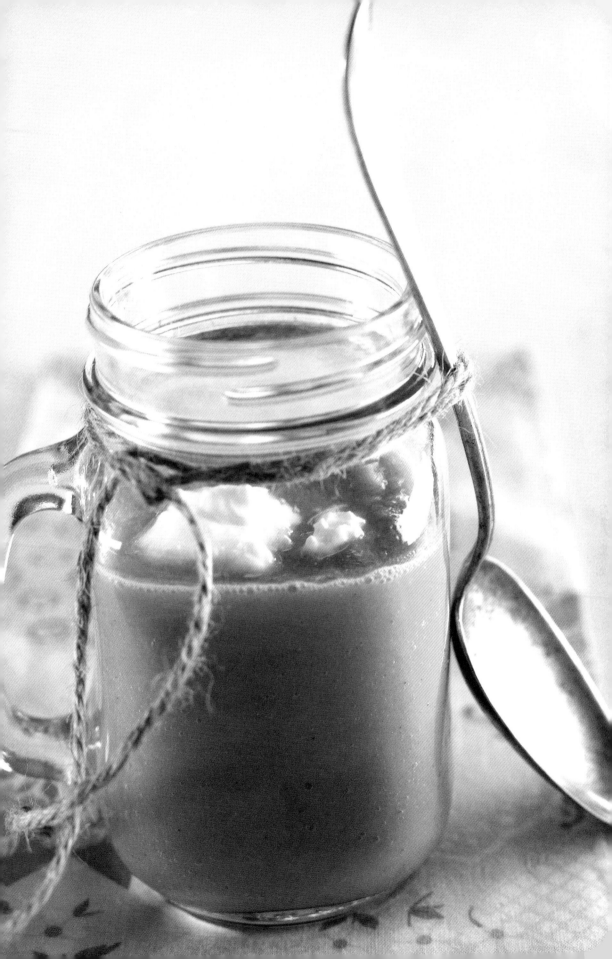

ASPARAGUS
SOUP

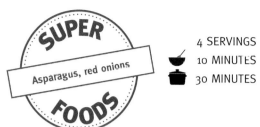

SUPER FOODS

Asparagus, red onions

4 SERVINGS

10 MINUTES

30 MINUTES

INGREDIENTS

2 tbsp olive oil

1 **red onion**, roughly chopped

2 cloves garlic, finely chopped

5 cups (1.25 liters) chicken or vegetable broth

3 tbsp quinoa, rinsed and drained

4 cups (1 liter) green **asparagus**, trimmed

4 tbsp chopped fresh cilantro

Seasoning to taste

METHOD

In a large saucepan, heat oil over medium heat and sauté onion and garlic for 3 to 5 minutes.

Add broth and quinoa and bring to a boil.

Add asparagus and continue cooking for 3 minutes. Reduce heat to medium-low. Cover and simmer for about 15 minutes.

Add cilantro, and blend mixture in a blender to consistency of soup.

Strain soup and season.

Nutrition Facts Per serving	
Amount	**% Daily Value**
Calories 160	
Fat 7 g	11%
Saturated 1 g	
+ Trans 0 g	
Polyunsaturated 1 g	
Omega-6 1 g	
Omega-3 0.1 g	
Monounsaturated 5 g	
Cholesterol 0 mg	0%
Sodium 110 mg	5%
Potassium 680 mg	20%
Carbohydrates 18 g	6%
Fiber 4 g	16%
Sugar 6 g	
Protein 7 g	
Vitamin A 146 ER	15%
Vitamin C 19 mg	30%
Calcium 59 mg	6%
Iron 2.6 mg	20%
Phosphorus 125.6 mg	10%

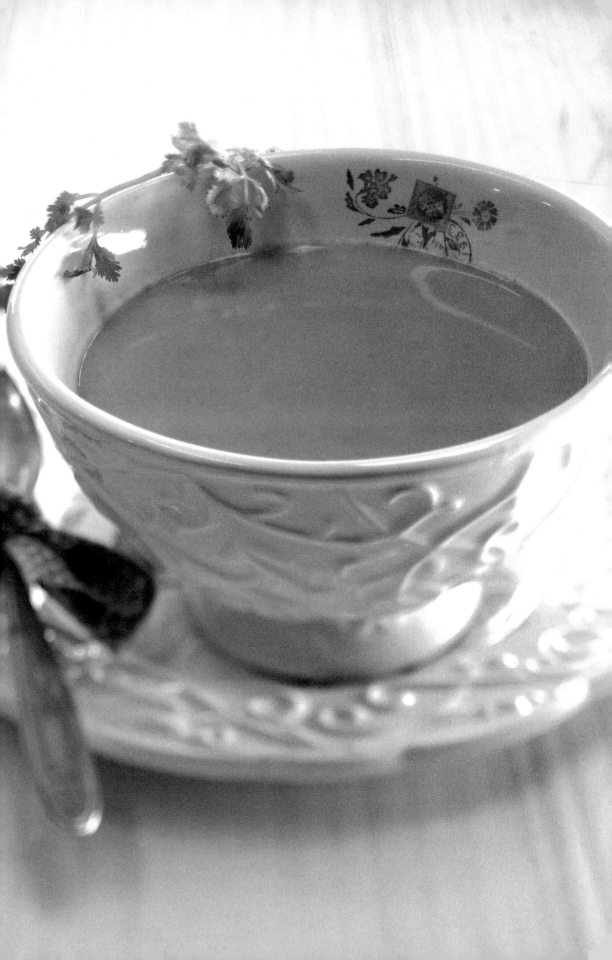

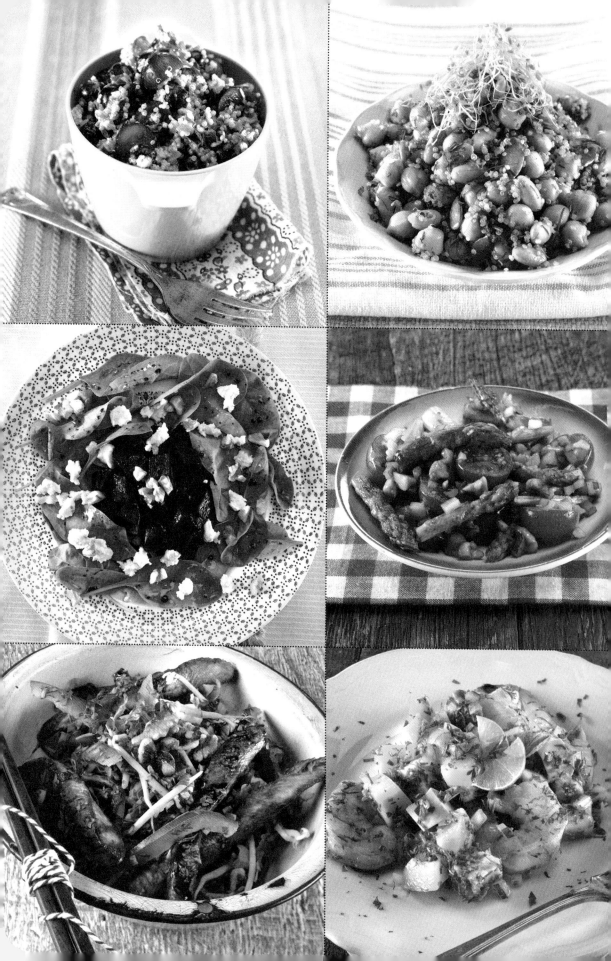

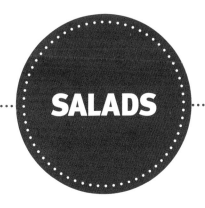

SALADS

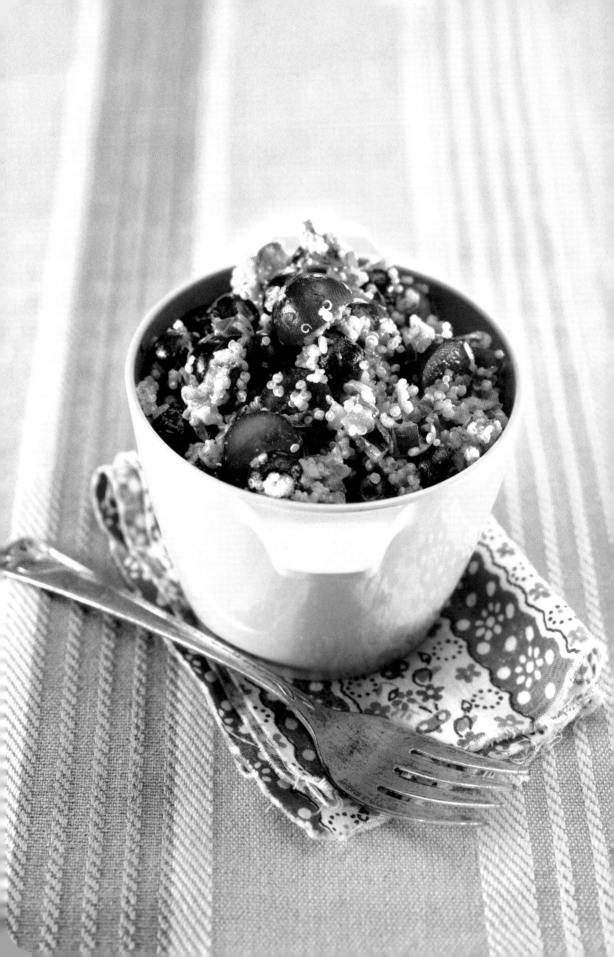

QUINOA SALAD WITH
RED GRAPES AND BLUEBERRIES

4 SERVINGS

15 MINUTES

15 MINUTES

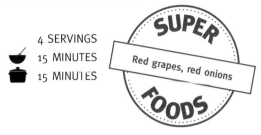

SUPER FOODS

Red grapes, red onions

INGREDIENTS

2 cups (500 ml) water

1 cup (250 ml) quinoa, rinsed and drained

1 cup (250 ml) fresh blueberries

1 cup (250 ml) **red grapes**, halved

1 **red onion**, finely chopped

3 tbsp chopped fresh cilantro

For the vinaigrette

1 tbsp olive oil

2 tbsp Dijon mustard

Juice of 1 lemon

1 clove garlic, finely chopped

1 tsp ground cumin

Seasoning to taste

METHOD

In a large saucepan over medium heat, bring water to a boil and then add quinoa. Reduce heat to low. Cover and simmer for 12 minutes. Drain and let cool.

In a salad bowl, combine quinoa, blueberries, grapes, onion and cilantro.

In a small bowl, combine ingredients for vinaigrette.

Pour vinaigrette over quinoa salad and toss.

Nutrition Facts Per serving	
Amount	**% Daily Value**
Calories 290	
Fat 6 g	9%
Saturated 1 g	
+ Trans 0 g	
Polyunsaturated 1.5 g	
Omega-6 1.5 g	
Omega-3 0.1 g	
Monounsaturated 3 g	
Cholesterol 0 mg	0%
Sodium 100 mg	4%
Potassium 600 mg	17%
Carbohydrates 51 g	17%
Fiber 6 g	24%
Sugar 13 g	
Protein 8 g	
Vitamin A 17 ER	2%
Vitamin C 28 mg	45%
Calcium 72 mg	6%
Iron 5.6 mg	40%
Phosphorus 219.4 mg	20%

CHEF'S TIP

To enjoy the full flavor of grapes, remove from the refrigerator at least 30 minutes before eating.

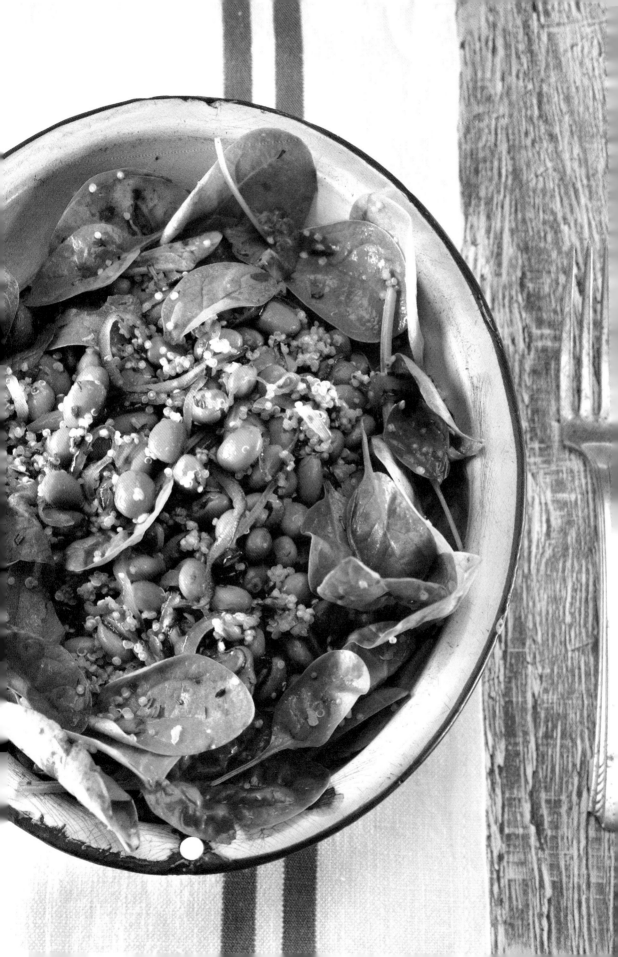

QUINOA SALAD WITH
PINTO BEANS AND SPINACH

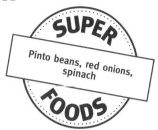

4 SERVINGS
10 MINUTES
20 MINUTES

Pinto beans, red onions, spinach

INGREDIENTS

½ cup (125 ml) water

¼ cup (60 ml) quinoa, rinsed and drained

2 tbsp olive oil

1 **red onion**, finely chopped

3 cloves garlic, finely chopped

1 can (19 oz/540 ml) **pinto beans**, drained and rinsed

1 cup (250 ml) baby **spinach**

1 tsp grated lemon zest

Juice of 2 lemons

2 tsp chopped fresh rosemary

¼ tsp crushed red pepper flakes

Seasoning to taste

METHOD

In a large saucepan over medium heat, bring water to a boil and then add quinoa. Reduce heat to low. Cover and simmer for 12 minutes. Drain and let cool.

In a skillet, heat oil over medium heat and sauté onion and garlic for 3 to 5 minutes. Let cool.

In a salad bowl, combine all ingredients and season.

Nutrition Facts Per serving	
Amount	**% Daily Value**
Calories 270	
Fat 8 g	12%
Saturated 1 g	
+ Trans 0 g	
Polyunsaturated 1.5 g	
Omega-6 1 g	
Omega-3 0.2 g	
Monounsaturated 5 g	
Cholesterol 0 mg	0%
Sodium 10 mg	0%
Potassium 580 mg	17%
Carbohydrates 39 g	13%
Fiber 8 g	32%
Sugar 3 g	
Protein 10 g	
Vitamin A 85 ER	8%
Vitamin C 22 mg	35%
Calcium 91 mg	8%
Iron 3.5 mg	25%
Phosphorus 192.3 mg	15%

CHICKPEA SALAD
WITH PUMPKIN SEEDS

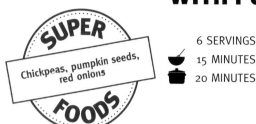

6 SERVINGS

15 MINUTES

20 MINUTES

INGREDIENTS

2 cups (500 ml) water

1 cup (250 ml) quinoa, rinsed and drained

1 cup (250 ml) frozen shelled edamame

4 tsp sesame oil

2 tsp balsamic vinegar

1 can (19 oz/540 ml) **chickpeas**, drained and rinsed

1 **red onion**, finely chopped

4 tbsp **pumpkin seeds**

4 tbsp chopped fresh dill

4 tbsp chopped fresh mint leaves

Alfalfa sprouts

Seasoning to taste

METHOD

In a large saucepan over medium heat, bring water to a boil and add quinoa. Reduce heat to low. Cover and simmer for 12 minutes. Drain and let cool.

Meanwhile, in another saucepan of boiling water over medium heat, cook edamame for 3 to 4 minutes. Let cool.

In a salad bowl, combine quinoa, edamame and remaining ingredients except alfalfa sprouts. Season and toss.

When ready to serve, garnish with alfalfa sprouts.

Nutrition Facts Per serving	
Amount	% Daily Value
Calories 360	
Fat 12 g	18%
Saturated 2 g	
+ Trans 0 g	
Polyunsaturated 4.5 g	
Omega-6 4.5 g	
Omega-3 0.1 g	
Monounsaturated 3.5 g	
Cholesterol 0 mg	0%
Sodium 120 mg	5%
Potassium 540 mg	15%
Carbohydrates 45 g	15%
Fiber 7 g	28%
Sugar 6 g	
Protein 17 g	
Vitamin A 32 ER	4%
Vitamin C 6 mg	10%
Calcium 92 mg	8%
Iron 7.4 mg	50%
Phosphorus 349.8 mg	30%

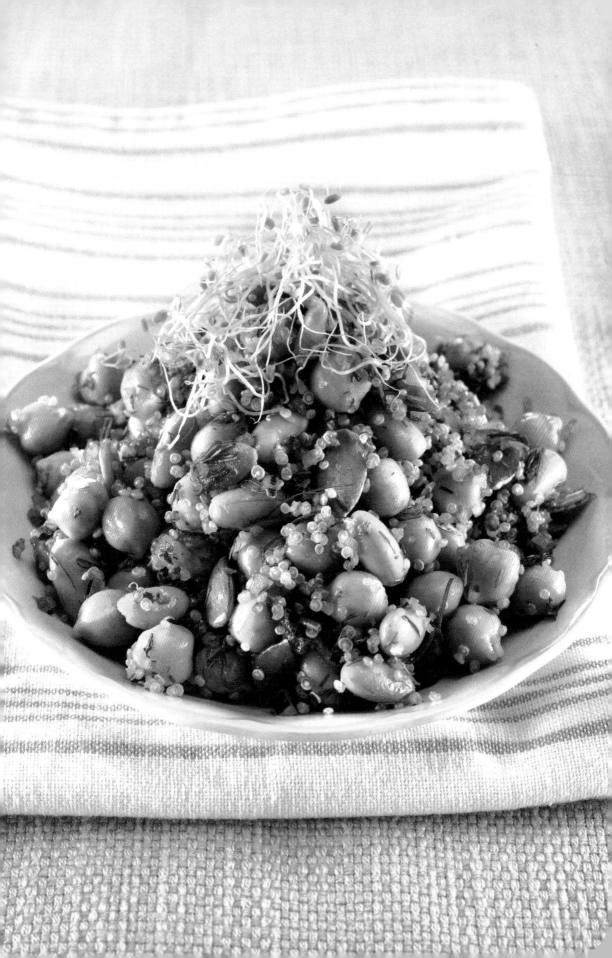

PINTO BEAN SALAD
WITH AVOCADO

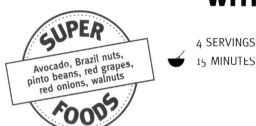

SUPER FOODS

Avocado, Brazil nuts, pinto beans, red grapes, red onions, walnuts

4 SERVINGS
15 MINUTES

INGREDIENTS

1 can (19 oz/540 ml) **pinto beans**, drained and rinsed

1 tsp balsamic vinegar

1 tbsp olive oil

Juice of 1 lime or 1 lemon

1 **avocado**, diced

1 cup (250 ml) cherry tomatoes, halved

10 **red grapes**, halved

3 tbsp coarsely chopped **walnuts** and **Brazil nuts**, mixed

1 **red onion**, finely chopped

1 clove garlic, finely chopped

½ cup (125 ml) chopped fresh cilantro

Seasoning to taste

METHOD

In a salad bowl, combine beans with vinegar. Let sit for at least 5 minutes.

Add remaining ingredients.

Toss well and adjust seasoning.

DID YOU KNOW?

The color of the avocado's skin depends on the variety and not ripeness. But avocados are definitely too ripe if the skin is dark near the stalk.

Nutrition Facts Per serving	
Amount	% Daily Value
Calories 310	
Fat 14 g	22%
Saturated 2.5 g	
+ Trans 0 g	
Polyunsaturated 3.5 g	
Omega-6 3 g	
Omega-3 0.5 g	
Monounsaturated 7 g	
Cholesterol 0 mg	0%
Sodium 20 mg	1%
Potassium 1070 mg	31%
Carbohydrates 37 g	12%
Fiber 11 g	44%
Sugar 7 g	
Protein 10 g	
Vitamin A 89 ER	8%
Vitamin C 74 mg	120%
Calcium 168 mg	15%
Iron 5.3 mg	40%
Phosphorus 199.3 mg	20%

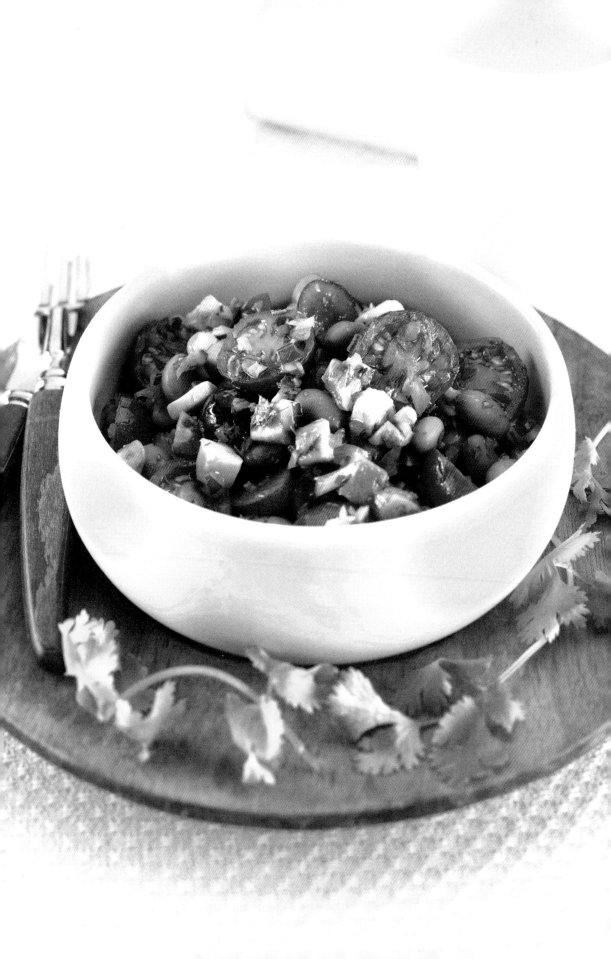

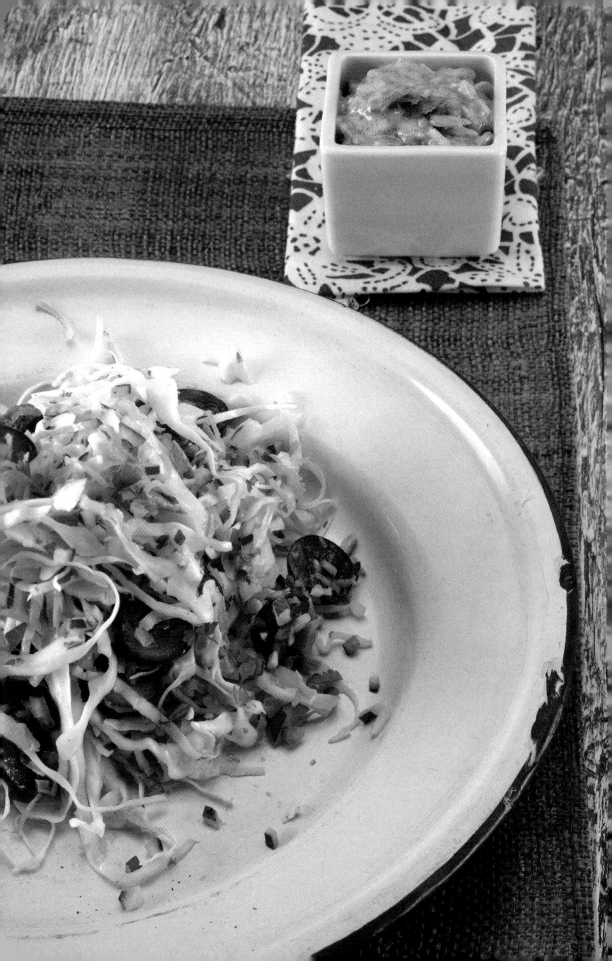

COLESLAW WITH GRAPES
AND SUNFLOWER SEEDS

4 SERVINGS

10 MINUTES

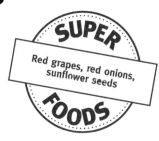

SUPER

Red grapes, red onions, sunflower seeds

FOODS

INGREDIENTS

1 small green cabbage, shredded

2 carrots, grated

1 small **red onion**, finely chopped

¼ cup (60 ml) chopped fresh cilantro

1 cup (250 ml) **red grapes**, halved

For the vinaigrette

3 tbsp olive oil

2 tbsp cider vinegar

2 tbsp Dijon mustard

Juice of 1 lemon

¼ cup (60 ml) **sunflower seeds**

Seasoning to taste

METHOD

In a salad bowl, combine cabbage, carrots, onion, cilantro and grapes.

In a small bowl, combine ingredients for vinaigrette.

When ready to serve, add vinaigrette to salad and toss gently.

Nutrition Facts Per serving	
Amount	% Daily Value
Calories 270	
Fat 15 g	23%
Saturated 2 g	
+ Trans 0 g	
Polyunsaturated 4.5 g	
Omega-6 4.5 g	
Omega-3 0.1 g	
Monounsaturated 8 g	
Cholesterol 0 mg	0%
Sodium 140 mg	11%
Potassium 790 mg	23%
Carbohydrates 28 g	9%
Fiber 6 g	24%
Sugar 15 g	
Protein 5 g	
Vitamin A 532 ER	50%
Vitamin C 77 mg	130%
Calcium 139 mg	15%
Iron 3.4 mg	25%
Phosphorus 180.4 mg	15%

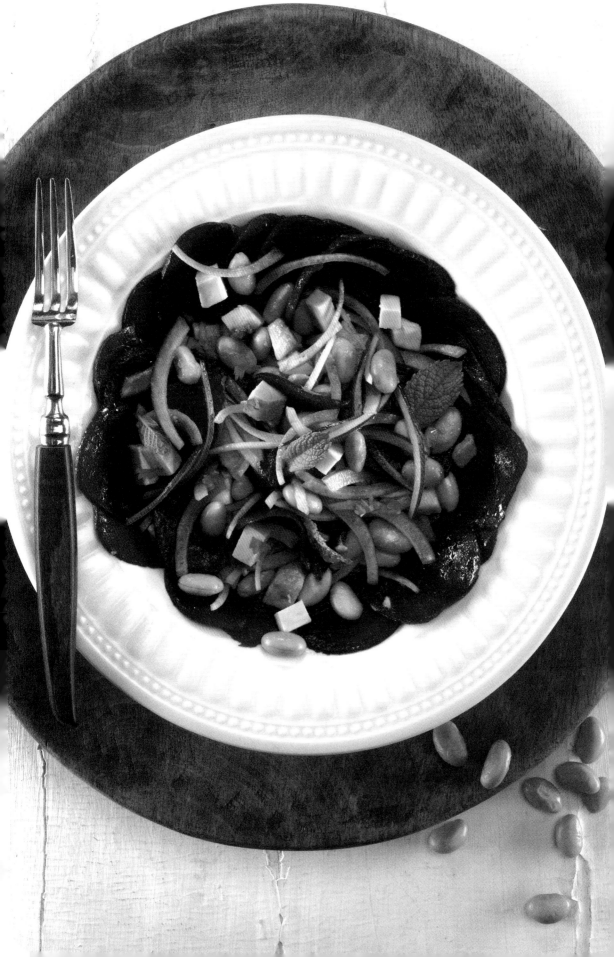

BEET SALAD WITH
AVOCADO AND EDAMAME

4 SERVINGS
20 MINUTES
1 HOUR

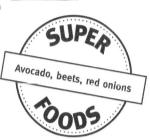

Avocado, beets, red onions

INGREDIENTS

4 medium **beets**, trimmed

1 cup (250 ml) frozen shelled edamame

2 medium **avocados**, cubed

1 small **red onion**, finely chopped

1 clove garlic, finely chopped

10 fresh mint leaves

1 tbsp chopped fresh cilantro

For the vinaigrette

4 tbsp olive oil

Juice of 1 lemon

½ tsp maple syrup

Seasoning to taste

METHOD

Position rack in center of oven and preheat to 350°F (180°C).

Wrap beets in aluminum foil. Place on a baking sheet and bake in center of preheated oven for 1 hour or until tip of a knife slides easily into beets. Let cool, then peel and slice.

Meanwhile, in a saucepan of boiling water over medium heat, blanch edamame for 3 to 4 minutes.

In a salad bowl, combine beets, edamame and remaining ingredients for salad.

In a small bowl, combine ingredients for vinaigrette.

Add vinaigrette to salad and toss.

Nutrition Facts Per serving	
Amount	**% Daily Value**
Calories 430	
Fat 31 g	48%
Saturated 5 g	
+ Trans 0 g	
Polyunsaturated 4 g	
Omega-6 3.5 g	
Omega-3 0.3 g	
Monounsaturated 18 g	
Cholesterol 0 mg	0%
Sodium 200 mg	8%
Potassium 760 mg	22%
Carbohydrates 26 g	9%
Fiber 12 g	48%
Sugar 10 g	
Protein 11 g	
Vitamin A 102 ER	10%
Vitamin C 27 mg	40%
Calcium 85 mg	8%
Iron 2.6 mg	20%
Phosphorus 92.2 mg	8%

BEET SALAD
WITH GOAT CHEESE

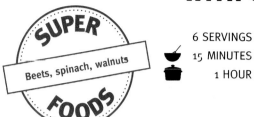

SUPER FOODS

Beets, spinach, walnuts

6 SERVINGS
15 MINUTES
1 HOUR

INGREDIENTS

8 medium **beets**, trimmed

4 cups (1 liter) baby **spinach** or arugula

⅓ cups (80 ml) coarsely chopped **walnuts**

¾ cup (180 ml) crumbled goat cheese

For the vinaigrette

2 tbsp olive oil

½ cup (125 ml) balsamic vinegar

2 tsp Dijon mustard

Seasoning to taste

METHOD

Position rack in center of oven and preheat to 350°F (180°C).

Wrap beets in aluminum foil. Place packages on a baking sheet and bake in center of preheated oven for 1 hour or until tip of a knife slides easily into beets. Let cool, then peel and cut in large cubes.

In a small bowl, emulsify oil, vinegar and mustard. Season.

In a bowl, combine beets and half the vinaigrette.

In another bowl, combine spinach and remaining vinaigrette.

Lay spinach on a serving platter, then garnish with beets, nuts and cheese.

Nutrition Facts Per serving	
Amount	**% Daily Value**
Calories 230	
Fat 16 g	25%
Saturated 6 g	
+ Trans 0 g	
Polyunsaturated 4 g	
Omega-6 3 g	
Omega-3 0.5 g	
Monounsaturated 5 g	
Cholesterol 20 mg	7%
Sodium 160 mg	7%
Potassium 360 mg	10%
Carbohydrates 12 g	4%
Fiber 2 g	8%
Sugar 9 g	
Protein 9 g	
Vitamin A 289 ER	30%
Vitamin C 8 mg	15%
Calcium 224 mg	20%
Iron 1.9 mg	15%
Phosphorus 204.2 mg	20%

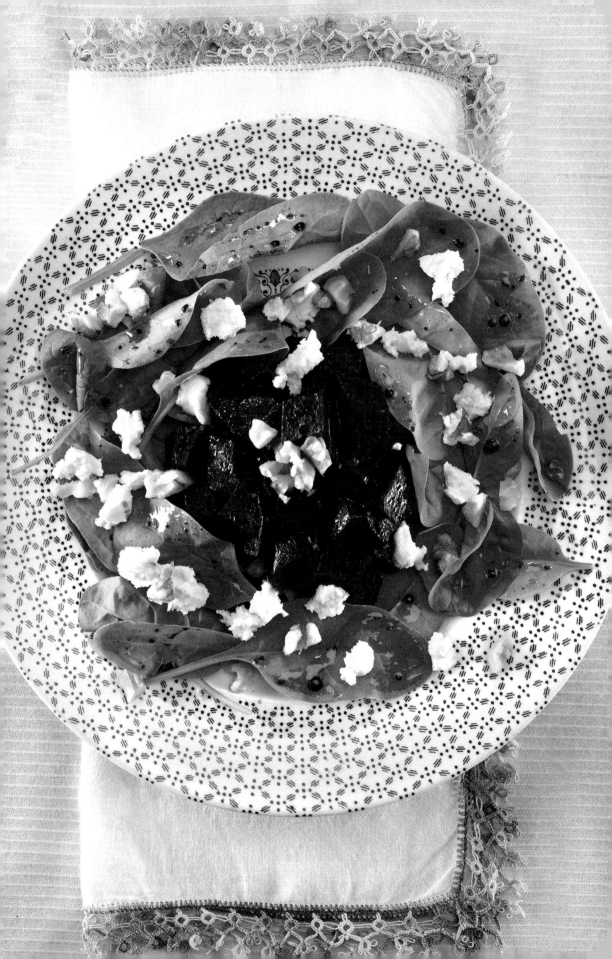

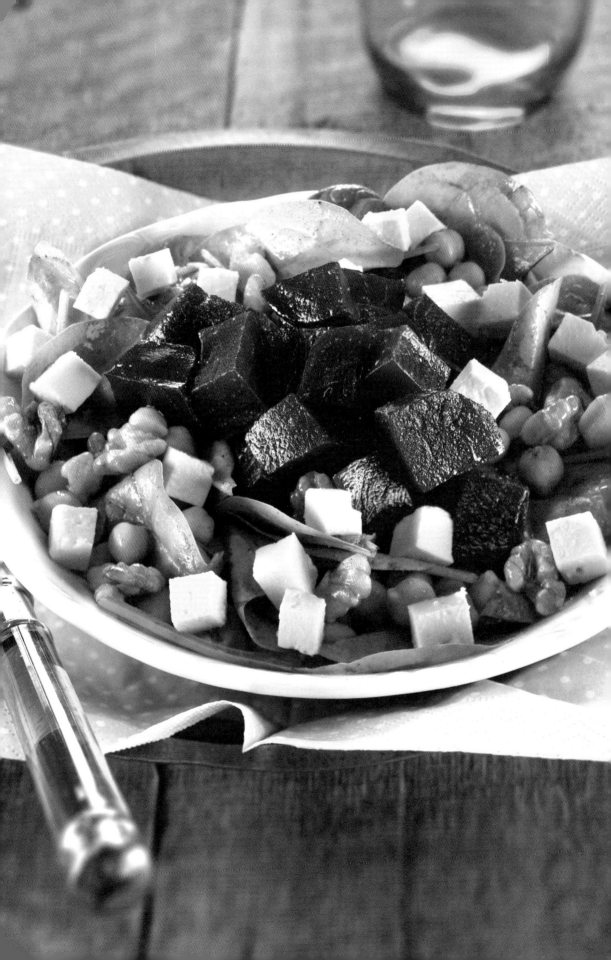

MEDLEY
SALAD

6 SERVINGS
15 MINUTES
1 HOUR

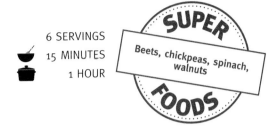

SUPER
FOODS

Beets, chickpeas, spinach, walnuts

INGREDIENTS

4 small **beets**, trimmed

Juice of 1 orange

1 tbsp olive oil

½ tsp ground cumin

3 cups (750 ml) baby **spinach**

1 can (19 oz/540 ml) **chickpeas**, drained and rinsed

½ cup (125 ml) **walnuts**

1¼ cups (300 ml) diced feta cheese

METHOD

Position rack in center of oven and preheat to 350°F (180°C).

Wrap beets in aluminum foil. Place packages on a baking sheet and bake in center of preheated oven for 1 hour or until tip of a knife slides easily into beets. Let cool, then peel and cut in cubes.

In a bowl, thoroughly combine beets with orange juice, oil and cumin.

In a salad bowl, place spinach, then add chickpeas, nuts and cheese. Top with beets.

Nutrition Facts Per serving	
Amount	**% Daily Value**
Calories 330	
Fat 20 g	31%
Saturated 7 g + Trans 0 g	
Polyunsaturated 6 g	
Omega-6 5 g	
Omega-3 1 g	
Monounsaturated 6 g	
Cholesterol 30 mg	10%
Sodium 410 mg	17%
Potassium 460 mg	13%
Carbohydrates 25 g	8%
Fiber 5 g	20%
Sugar 9 g	
Protein 13 g	
Vitamin A 189 ER	20%
Vitamin C 14 mg	25%
Calcium 228 mg	20%
Iron 3.2 mg	25%
Phosphorus 275.2 mg	25%

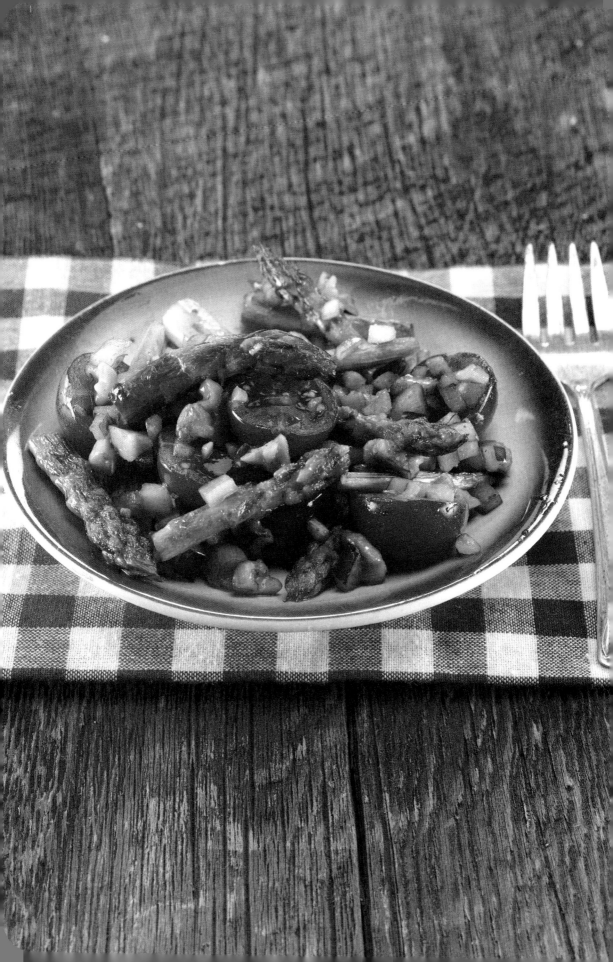

ASPARAGUS SALAD
WITH WALNUTS

4 SERVINGS
10 MINUTES
5 MINUTES

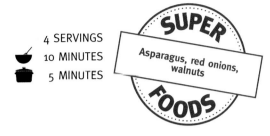

SUPER
FOODS

Asparagus, red onions, walnuts

INGREDIENTS

2 tbsp olive oil, divided

24 green **asparagus**, trimmed and cut in sections

½ cup (125 ml) coarsely chopped **walnuts**

2 tbsp balsamic vinegar

1 **red onion**, finely chopped

15 cherry tomatoes, halved

Seasoning to taste

METHOD

In a hot skillet, heat 1 tbsp of oil over low heat and cook asparagus and nuts for 3 to 5 minutes.

Meanwhile, combine remaining ingredients and 1 tbsp of oil in a salad bowl.

Add asparagus and nuts. Gently combine so as not to break asparagus. Adjust seasoning.

Nutrition Facts Per serving	
Amount	**% Daily Value**
Calories 230	
Fat 17 g	26%
Saturated 2 g	
+ Trans 0 g	
Polyunsaturated 8 g	
Omega-6 6 g	
Omega-3 1.5 g	
Monounsaturated 6 g	
Cholesterol 0 mg	0%
Sodium 20 mg	1%
Potassium 440 mg	13%
Carbohydrates 13 g	4%
Fiber 4 g	16%
Sugar 6 g	
Protein 5 g	
Vitamin A 16 ER	15%
Vitamin C 133 mg	25%
Calcium 51 mg	4%
Iron 1.6 mg	10%
Phosphorus 122.9 mg	10%

RAW ASPARAGUS
SALAD

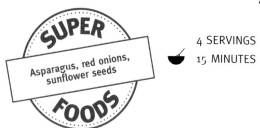

SUPER FOODS

Asparagus, red onions, sunflower seeds

4 SERVINGS
15 MINUTES

INGREDIENTS

12 green **asparagus,** trimmed

2 tbsp olive oil

Juice of 1 lime or 1 lemon

2 tsp Dijon mustard

1 small **red onion,** diced

½ cup (125 ml) freshly grated Parmesan

2 tbsp **sunflower seeds**

2 tbsp pine nuts

Seasoning to taste

METHOD

Cut tips off asparagus and grate stalks in thin strips using a vegetable peeler.

In a salad bowl, combine asparagus tips and stalks with remaining ingredients.

COMMON MISCONCEPTIONS
Eating asparagus harms kidneys.

FALSE. When you eat asparagus, your urine may give off an odor because of the presence of strong smelling sulfur derivatives. This minor annoyance in no way means the kidneys aren't functioning properly. But asparagus is a diuretic. It promotes the production and elimination of urine, accelerating the evacuation of waste.

Nutrition Facts Per serving	
Amount	**% Daily Value**
Calories 180	
Fat 14 g	22%
Saturated 3.5 g	
+ Trans 0 g	
Polyunsaturated 3.5 g	
Omega-6 3.5 g	
Omega-3 0.3 g	
Monounsaturated 7 g	
Cholesterol 10 mg	3%
Sodium 220 mg	9%
Potassium 190 mg	5%
Carbohydrates 7 g	2%
Fiber 2 g	8%
Sugar 2 g	
Protein 7 g	
Vitamin A 50 ER	6%
Vitamin C 10 mg	15%
Calcium 162 mg	15%
Iron 1.5 mg	10%
Phosphorus 179 mg	15%

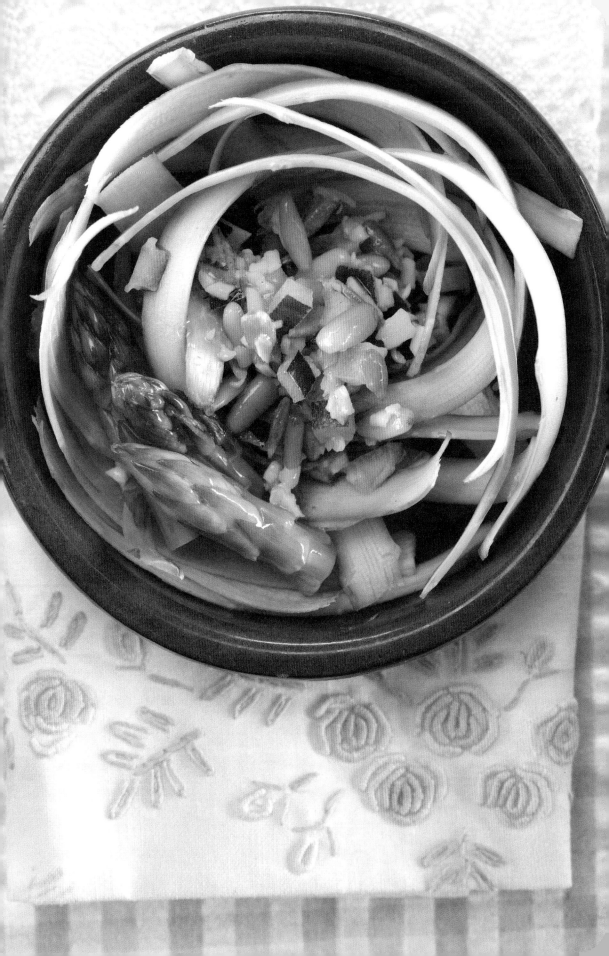

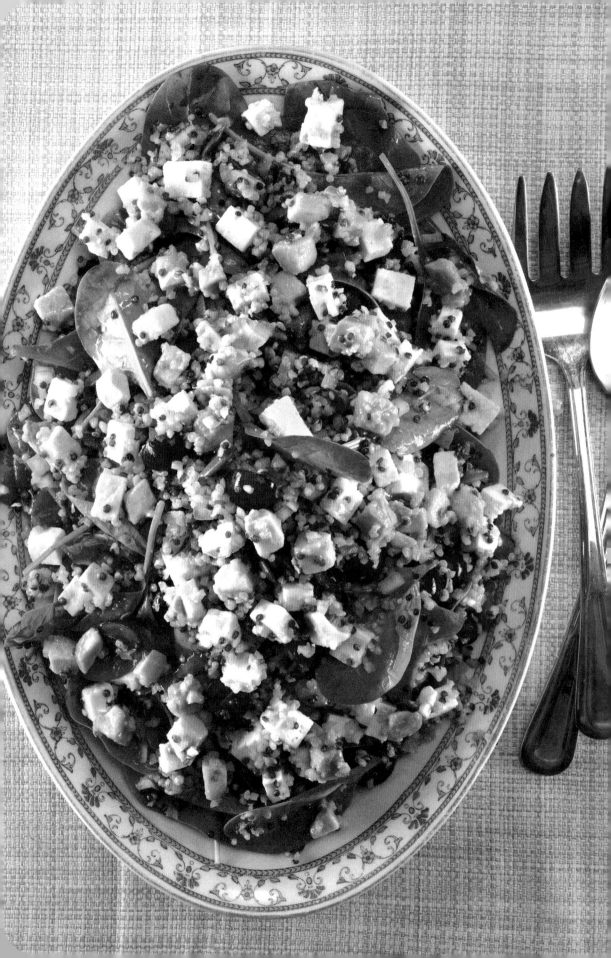

RAINBOW
SALAD

6 SERVINGS
10 MINUTES
15 MINUTES

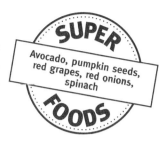

SUPER FOODS

Avocado, pumpkin seeds, red grapes, red onions, spinach

INGREDIENTS

2 cups (500 ml) water

1 cup (250 ml) quinoa, rinsed and drained

1 small **red onion**, finely chopped

1 **avocado**, diced

2 cups (500 ml) baby **spinach**

1 cup (250 ml) **red grapes**, halved

⅔ cup (160 ml) diced feta cheese

4 tbsp **pumpkin seeds**

For the vinaigrette

¼ cup (60 ml) olive oil

Juice of 1 lemon

Seasoning to taste

METHOD

In large saucepan over medium heat, bring water to a boil and add quinoa. Reduce heat to low. Cover and simmer for 12 minutes. Drain and let cool.

In a salad bowl, thoroughly combine quinoa with remaining salad ingredients.

In a small bowl, combine ingredients for vinaigrette.

Add vinaigrette to salad and toss.

Nutrition Facts Per serving	
Amount	**% Daily Value**
Calories 390	
Fat 23 g	35%
Saturated 6 g	
+ Trans 0 g	
Polyunsaturated 4.5 g	
Omega-6 4 g	
Omega-3 0.2 g	
Monounsaturated 12 g	
Cholesterol 15 mg	5%
Sodium 200 mg	9%
Potassium 630 mg	18%
Carbohydrates 34 g	11%
Fiber 6 g	24%
Sugar 8 g	
Protein 11 g	
Vitamin A 128 ER	15%
Vitamin C 22 mg	35%
Calcium 125 mg	10%
Iron 4.8 mg	35%
Phosphorus 325.7 mg	30%

NIÇOISE SALAD WITH
SARDINES AND SPINACH

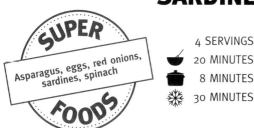

4 SERVINGS

20 MINUTES

8 MINUTES

30 MINUTES

INGREDIENTS

8 green **asparagus**, trimmed and cut in sections

5 cups (1.25 liters) baby **spinach**

1 small **red onion**, finely chopped

10 cherry tomatoes

6 black olives, halved

2 large hard-boiled **eggs**, sliced

2 cans (each 3.5 oz/100 g) **sardines** in olive oil or water, drained

For the vinaigrette

2 tbsp olive oil

2 tbsp balsamic vinegar

1 tsp old-fashioned mustard

1 clove garlic, finely chopped

¼ tsp dried tarragon

Seasoning to taste

METHOD

In a steamer basket over medium heat, cook asparagus for 8 minutes.

In a salad bowl, combine ingredients for salad, except eggs and sardines.

In a small bowl, combine ingredients for vinaigrette.

Add vinaigrette to salad and toss.

Arrange eggs and sardines on salad and refrigerate for 30 minutes to allow flavors to develop.

Nutrition Facts Per serving	
Amount	**% Daily Value**
Calories 240	
Fat 16 g	25%
Saturated 3.5 g	
+ Trans 0 g	
Polyunsaturated 2.5 g	
Omega-6 1.5 g	
Omega-3 1 g	
Monounsaturated 10 g	
Cholesterol 125 mg	42%
Sodium 490 mg	21%
Potassium 610 mg	17%
Carbohydrates 9 g	3%
Fiber 3 g	12%
Sugar 4 g	
Protein 16 g	
Vitamin A 478 ER	50%
Vitamin C 20 mg	35%
Calcium 211 mg	20%
Iron 3.8 mg	25%
Phosphorus 267.4 mg	25%

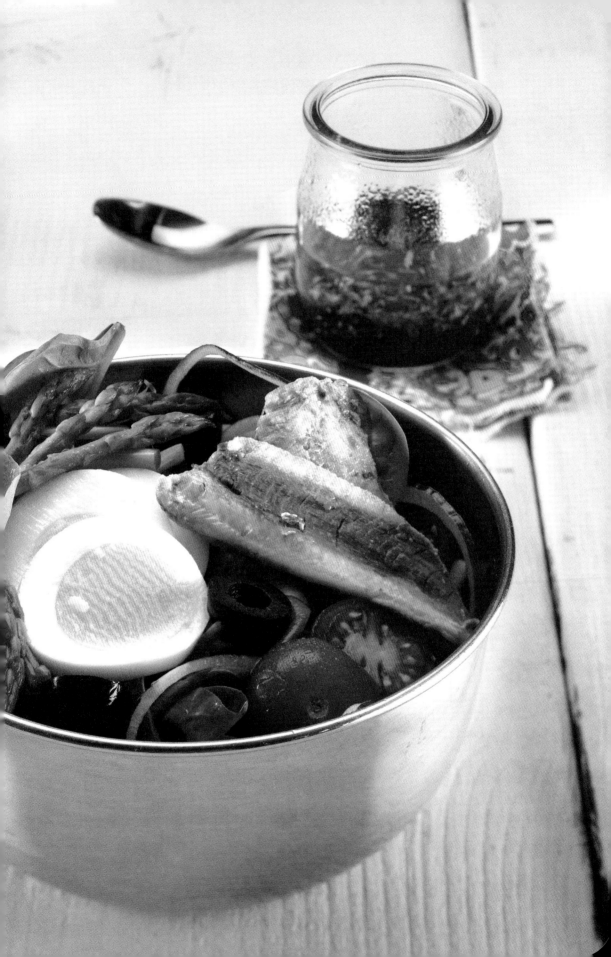

GREEK SALAD WITH CHICKPEAS
AND SARDINES

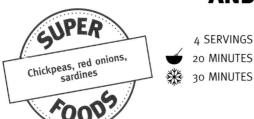

SUPER FOODS

Chickpeas, red onions, sardines

4 SERVINGS

20 MINUTES

30 MINUTES

INGREDIENTS

3 medium tomatoes, in chunks

1 cucumber, diced

1 can (19 oz/540 ml) **chickpeas**, drained and rinsed

1 small **red onion**, finely chopped

2 tbsp Kalamata olives, sliced in rounds

⅔ cup (160 ml) crumbled feta cheese

2 cans (each 3.5 oz/100 g) **sardines** in olive oil or water, drained

For the vinaigrette

2 tbsp olive oil

Juice of 1 lemon

2 cloves garlic, finely chopped

2 tbsp chopped fresh parsley

2 tsp dried oregano

Seasoning to taste

METHOD

In a salad bowl, combine ingredients for salad, except sardines.

In a small bowl, combine ingredients for vinaigrette.

Add vinaigrette to salad and refrigerate for 30 minutes to allow flavors to develop.

Toss salad and top with sardines.

Nutrition Facts Per serving		
Amount		**% Daily Value**
Calories 430		
Fat 20 g		31%
Saturated 6 g		
+ Trans 0 g		
Polyunsaturated 3 g		
Omega-6 2 g		
Omega-3 1 g		
Monounsaturated 10 g		
Cholesterol 55 mg		18%
Sodium 540 mg		22%
Potassium 880 mg		25%
Carbohydrates 39 g		13%
Fiber 7 g		28%
Sugar 11 g		
Protein 24 g		
Vitamin A 160 ER		15%
Vitamin C 35 mg		60%
Calcium 337 mg		30%
Iron 5.2 mg		35%
Phosphorus 476 mg		45%

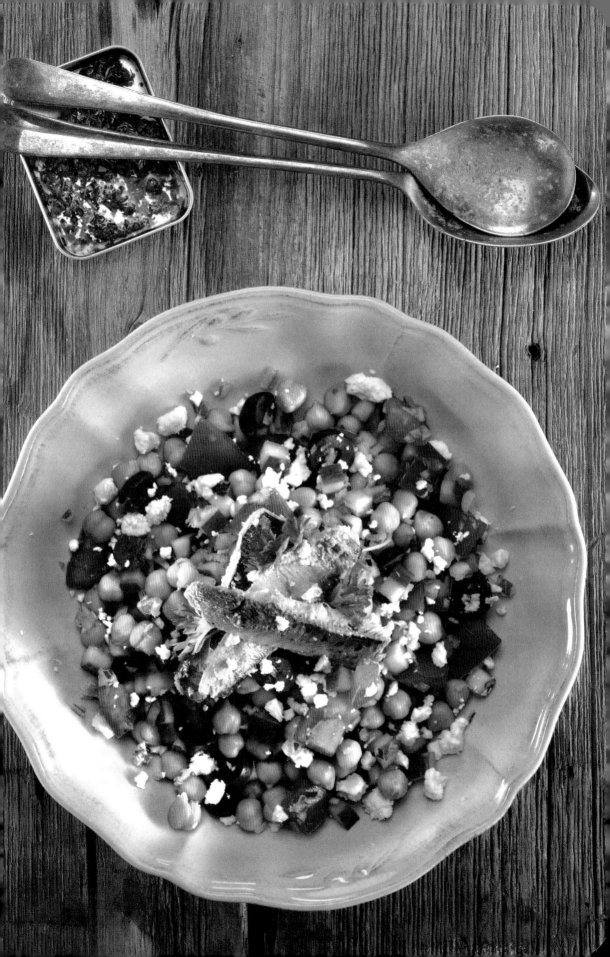

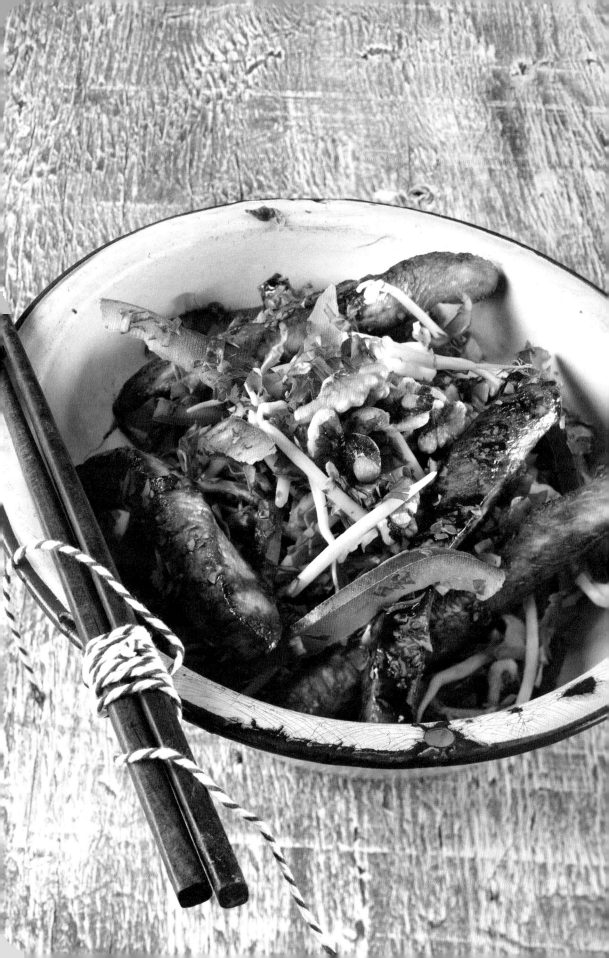

WARM ASIAN
CHICKEN SALAD

4 SERVINGS
15 MINUTES
20 MINUTES

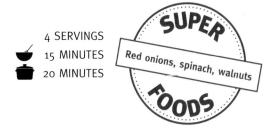

Red onions, spinach, walnuts

SUPER FOODS

INGREDIENTS

1 tbsp sesame or olive oil

1 small **red onion**, finely chopped

2 cloves garlic, finely chopped

2 tbsp finely chopped fresh ginger

1 lb (454 g) boneless, skinless chicken breast or thighs, in thin strips

⅔ cup (160 ml) chicken or vegetable broth

3 tbsp low-sodium soy sauce

1 to 2 tsp honey or maple syrup

4 cups (1 liter) baby **spinach**, chopped

1 large red pepper, in thin strips

1½ cups (375 ml) bean sprouts

¼ cup (60 ml) **walnuts**

¼ cup (60 ml) chopped fresh parsley

METHOD

In a skillet, heat oil over medium heat and sauté onion, garlic and ginger for 3 to 5 minutes. Add chicken and continue cooking for about 10 minutes.

Meanwhile, in a bowl, combine broth, soy sauce and honey. Pour into skillet and cook, stirring, for 2 minutes or until sauce thickens.

In a salad bowl, combine spinach, pepper and bean sprouts.

When ready to serve, arrange chicken on the spinach mixture and top with nuts and parsley.

Nutrition Facts Per serving	
Amount	% Daily Value
Calories 350	
Fat 18 g	28%
Saturated 3.5 g + Trans 0 g	
Polyunsaturated 7 g	
Omega-6 6 g	
Omega-3 1 g	
Monounsaturated 6 g	
Cholesterol 85 mg	28%
Sodium 530 mg	22%
Potassium 740 mg	21%
Carbohydrates 13 g	4%
Fiber 2 g	8%
Sugar 5 g	
Protein 35 g	
Vitamin A 385 ER	40%
Vitamin C 27 mg	45%
Calcium 84 mg	8%
Iron 3.6 mg	25%
Phosphorus 331.5 mg	30%

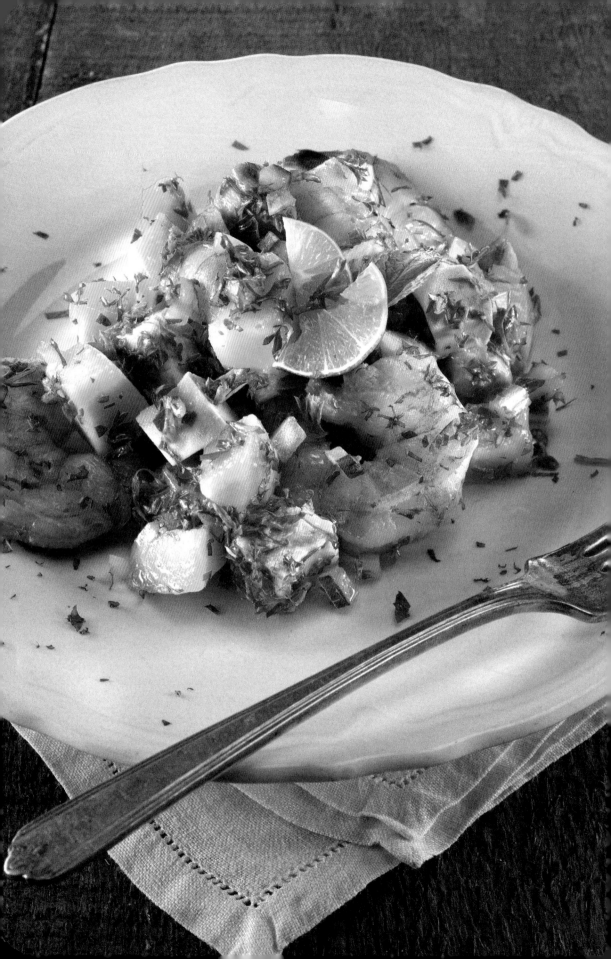

SHRIMP SALAD WITH AVOCADO
AND MANGO

🍜 4 SERVINGS
15 MINUTES

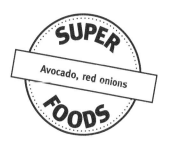

SUPER
FOODS

Avocado, red onions

INGREDIENTS

1 tbsp olive oil

Juice of 1 lime or 1 lemon

1 tsp honey or maple syrup

2 tbsp finely chopped **red onion**

½ cup (125 ml) finely chopped fresh parsley

2 tbsp chopped fresh mint leaves

½ tsp crushed red pepper flakes

2 **avocados**, diced

2 mangos, diced

1 lb (454 g) large cooked shrimp, peeled

Seasoning to taste

METHOD

In a salad bowl, gently combine all ingredients.

Nutrition Facts Per serving	
Amount	**% Daily Value**
Calories 430	
Fat 20 g	31%
Saturated 4 g + Trans 0 g	
Polyunsaturated 3.5 g	
Omega-6 3 g	
Omega-3 0.5 g	
Monounsaturated 11 g	
Cholesterol 220 mg	73%
Sodium 270 mg	11%
Potassium 1000 mg	29%
Carbohydrates 34 g	11%
Fiber 11 g	44%
Sugar 21 g	
Protein 28 g	
Vitamin A 270 ER	25%
Vitamin C 36 mg	60%
Calcium 90 mg	8%
Iron 4.8 mg	35%
Phosphorus 238.7 mg	20%

DID YOU KNOW?

Avocados can stay up to six months on the branch without going bad, and they ripen only once picked. Ripening takes just a few days.

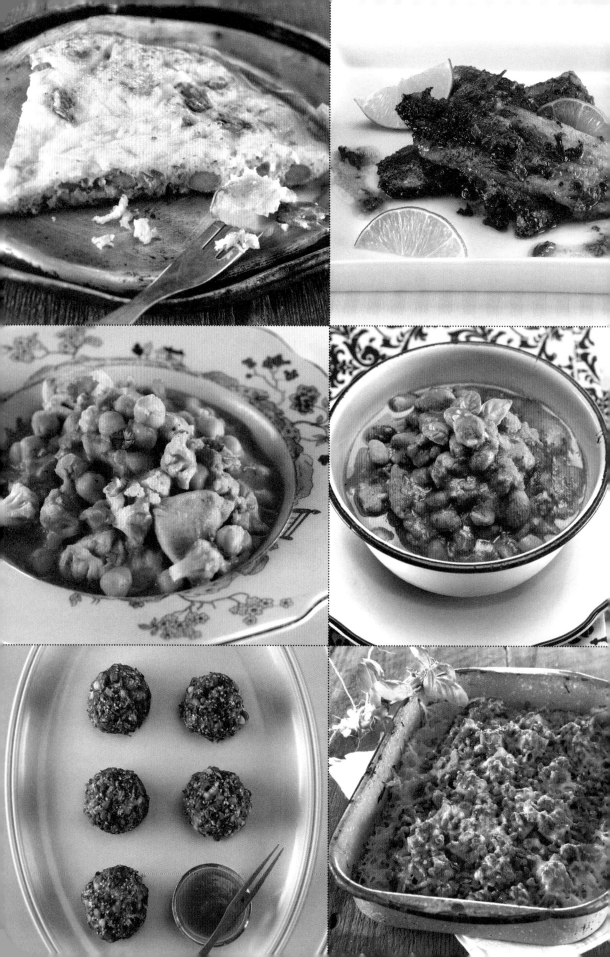

MAIN COURSES

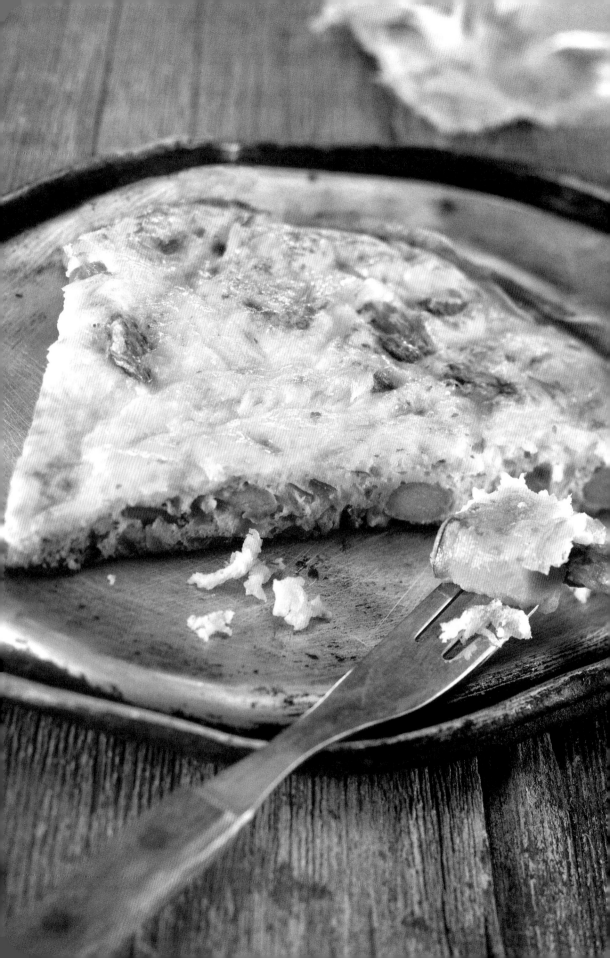

ASPARAGUS AND SWEET POTATO
FRITTATA

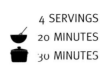

🥄 4 SERVINGS
   20 MINUTES
🍲 30 MINUTES

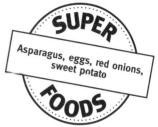

SUPER FOODS

Asparagus, eggs, red onions, sweet potato

INGREDIENTS

2 tbsp olive oil

1 **red onion**, finely chopped

1 **sweet potato**, unpeeled, washed and diced

12 green **asparagus**, trimmed and cut in 1-inch (2.5 cm) sections

3 cloves garlic, finely chopped

8 large **eggs**, beaten

¼ cup (60 ml) 2% milk, or lighter

¼ cup (60 ml) grated Parmesan

4 tbsp chopped fresh parsley

Pinch cayenne pepper

1 cup (250 ml) grated mozzarella

Seasoning to taste

METHOD

In an ovenproof skillet, heat oil over medium heat and sauté onion and sweet potato for 6 to 7 minutes or until they are browned on all sides.

Add asparagus and garlic. Cook, stirring often, for 3 to 5 minutes or until asparagus is tender, but still crisp.

Meanwhile, in a large bowl, combine eggs, milk, Parmesan, parsley and cayenne pepper.

In a lightly oiled skillet over medium-low heat, add egg mixture and combine quickly. Top with cheese and cook, without stirring, for 10 to 12 minutes or until eggs are almost set.

Place skillet under preheated oven broiler for 1 to 3 minutes or until top of frittata is golden.

Let sit for 5 minutes. Cut in four equal pieces and serve.

COMMON MISCONCEPTIONS
Eating eggs increases cholesterol.
FALSE. Old beliefs die hard. Scientific research shows that dietary cholesterol, such as the cholesterol found in eggs, has very little impact on blood cholesterol levels.

Nutrition Facts Per serving		
Amount		**% Daily Value**
Calories 390		
Fat 25 g		38%
Saturated 9 g		
+ Trans 0.2 g		
Polyunsaturated 2.5 g		
Omega-6 2 g		
Omega-3 0.2 g		
Monounsaturated 10 g		
Cholesterol 400 mg		133%
Sodium 460 mg		19%
Potassium 450 mg		13%
Carbohydrates 16 g		5%
Fiber 3 g		12%
Sugar 6 g		
Protein 25 g		
Vitamin A 758 ER		80%
Vitamin C 13 mg		20%
Calcium 382 mg		35%
Iron 2.2 mg		15%
Phosphorus 248.8 mg		25%

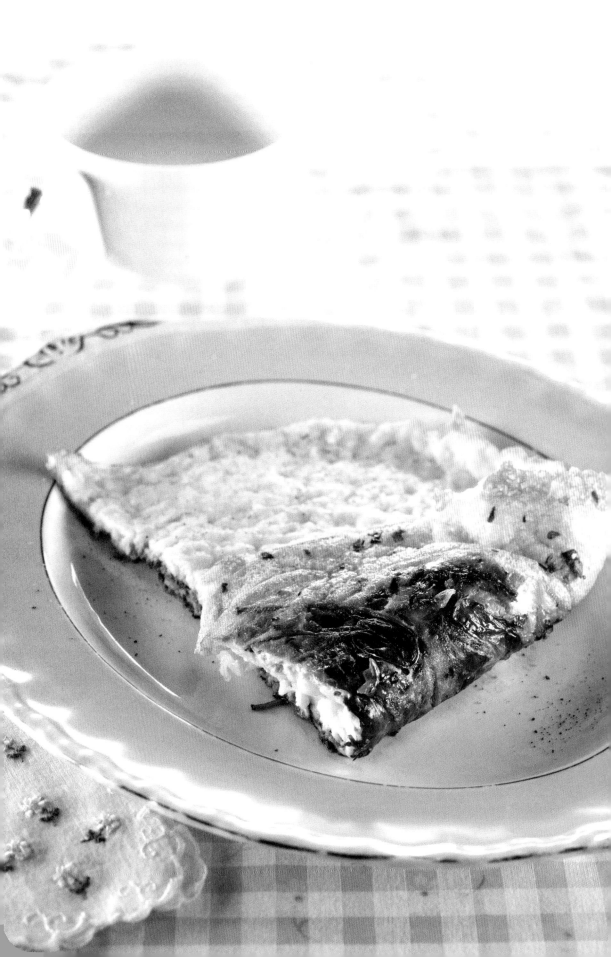

CHEESE AND SPINACH
OMELET

2 SERVINGS
5 MINUTES
10 MINUTES

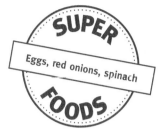

Eggs, red onions, spinach

INGREDIENTS

1 tbsp olive oil

1 small **red onion**, finely chopped

2 cloves garlic, finely chopped

Pinch crushed red pepper flakes

1 cup (250 ml) baby **spinach**

4 **egg** whites, beaten to form peaks

4 **egg** yolks, beaten

1 cup (250 ml) grated 20% M.F. cheese, or lighter

METHOD

In a skillet, heat oil over medium heat and sauté onion and garlic for 3 to 5 minutes. Add chiles and cook for 1 minute. Add spinach and continue cooking a few minutes. Reserve.

In a bowl, using a spatula, fold in egg whites and yolks until texture is smooth.

Pour egg mixture over spinach and top with cheese. Cook for 3 to 5 minutes or until omelet is set.

Nutrition Facts Per serving	
Amount	**% Daily Value**
Calories 370	
Fat 26 g	40%
Saturated 10 g	
+ Trans 0.4 g	
Polyunsaturated 2.5 g	
Omega-6 2 g	
Omega-3 0.2 g	
Monounsaturated 12 g	
Cholesterol 410 mg	135%
Sodium 420 mg	18%
Potassium 310 mg	9%
Carbohydrates 7 g	2%
Fiber 1 g	4%
Sugar 3 g	
Protein 28 g	
Vitamin A 359 ER	35%
Vitamin C 7 mg	10%
Calcium 465 mg	40%
Iron 1.8 mg	15%
Phosphorus 440.9 mg	40%

SMOKED SALMON POACHED EGGS ON A BED
OF GRILLED ASPARAGUS

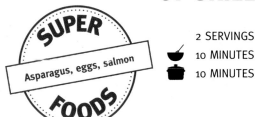

SUPER
Asparagus, eggs, salmon
FOODS

2 SERVINGS
10 MINUTES
10 MINUTES

INGREDIENTS

2 large **eggs**

8 green **asparagus**, trimmed

2 tbsp olive oil

2 oz (60 g) smoked **salmon**

Seasoning to taste

METHOD

In a small saucepan over high heat, bring lightly salted water to a boil, then reduce heat to low.

In a small bowl, break an egg and slide it into the water. Repeat with second egg. Cook eggs for 2 to 3 minutes or until desired doneness. Remove eggs with a skimmer and reserve on paper towel.

Meanwhile, preheat oven broiler and uniformly distribute asparagus on a baking sheet. Pour oil over top and season. Cook under preheated broiler, turning partway through cooking, for 5 to 6 minutes or until tender.

Distribute asparagus on plates. Place a poached egg on top and garnish with smoked salmon, leaving tip of asparagus bare. Season.

DID YOU KNOW?

In its wild state, salmon feeds on shellfish. Their carotenoid orange pigment is retained by the fish's muscle tissue, which gives the flesh its color, ranging from pale pink to bright red, depending on the variety. When salmon is farmed, fish farmers put synthetic coloring in their food to give the salmon flesh its characteristic color. The omega-3s found in salmon come from the algae they eat.

Nutrition Facts Per serving	
Amount	**% Daily Value**
Calories 240	
Fat 19 g	29%
Saturated 3.5 g	
+ Trans 0 g	
Polyunsaturated 2.5 g	
Omega-6 2 g	
Omega-3 0.3 g	
Monounsaturated 12 g	
Cholesterol 190 mg	65%
Sodium 300 mg	13%
Potassium 250 mg	7%
Carbohydrates 3 g	1%
Fiber 1 g	4%
Sugar 1 g	
Protein 13 g	
Vitamin A 138 ER	15%
Vitamin C 5 mg	8%
Calcium 42 mg	4%
Iron 1.4 mg	10%
Phosphorus 148.3 mg	15%

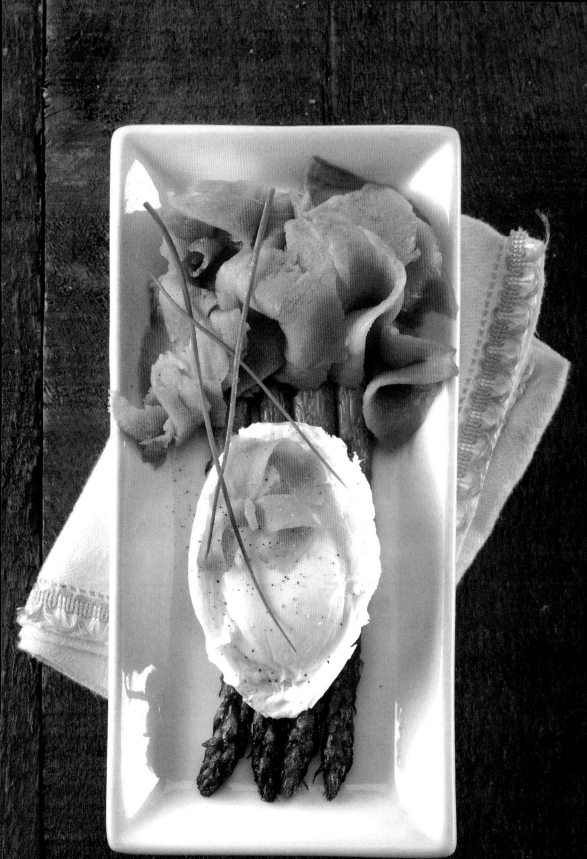

CARPE DIEM SALMON WITH
ASPARAGUS AND AVOCADO

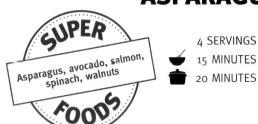

4 SERVINGS
15 MINUTES
20 MINUTES

INGREDIENTS

4 **salmon** fillets, each 3 to 4 oz (90 to 120 g), cut in half widthwise

2 red peppers, halved and seeded

1 tbsp olive oil

12 green **asparagus**, trimmed and cut in sections

2 cups (500 ml) baby **spinach**

1 **avocado**, sliced

2 tbsp **Spinach** and **Walnut** Pesto (see recipe p. 90) or store-bought basil pesto

Seasoning to taste

METHOD

Preheat oven to 400°F (200°C).

Season salmon fillets with salt and pepper.

Place peppers on an oiled baking sheet, skin side up, and bake in preheated oven for about 20 minutes or until they start to wrinkle.

After 10 minutes of cooking, place salmon fillets on baking sheet. Bake with peppers for about 8 minutes.

Meanwhile, in a skillet, heat oil over medium heat and sauté asparagus for about 3 minutes. Add spinach and wilt for 2 minutes.

Flatten peppers into a rectangle. Place a salmon fillet on each half pepper. Distribute spinach, asparagus and avocado on top. Cover each portion with a fillet. Garnish with pesto and season.

Nutrition Facts Per serving	
Amount	**% Daily Value**
Calories 340	
Fat 23 g	35%
Saturated 4 g	
+ Trans 0.1 g	
Polyunsaturated 5 g	
Omega-6 3 g	
Omega-3 2 g	
Monounsaturated 9 g	
Cholesterol 60 mg	20%
Sodium 105 mg	4%
Potassium 800 mg	23%
Carbohydrates 9 g	3%
Fiber 5 g	20%
Sugar 3 g	
Protein 23 g	
Vitamin A 324 ER	30%
Vitamin C 45 mg	75%
Calcium 56 mg	6%
Iron 1.4 mg	10%
Phosphorus 294.3 mg	25%

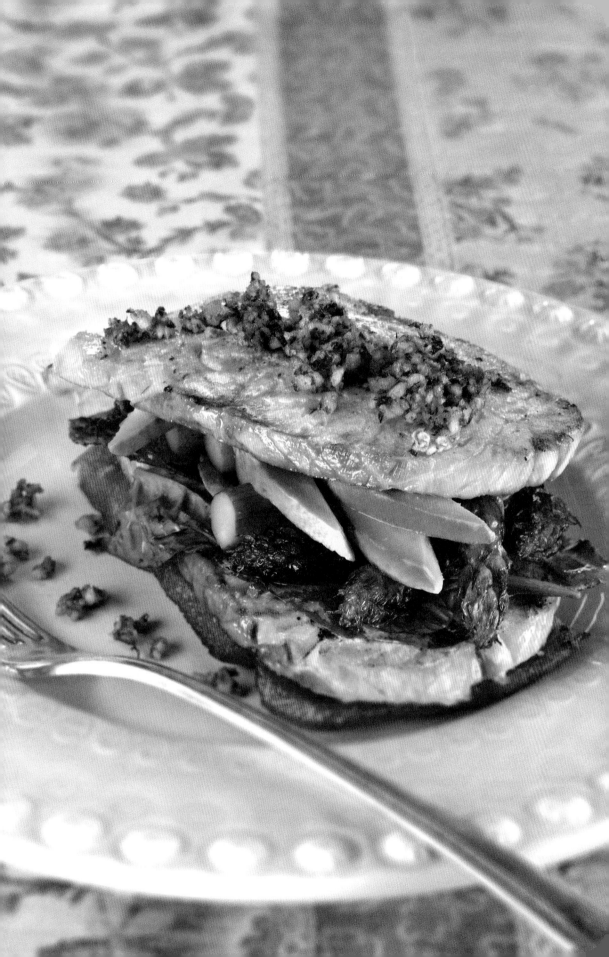

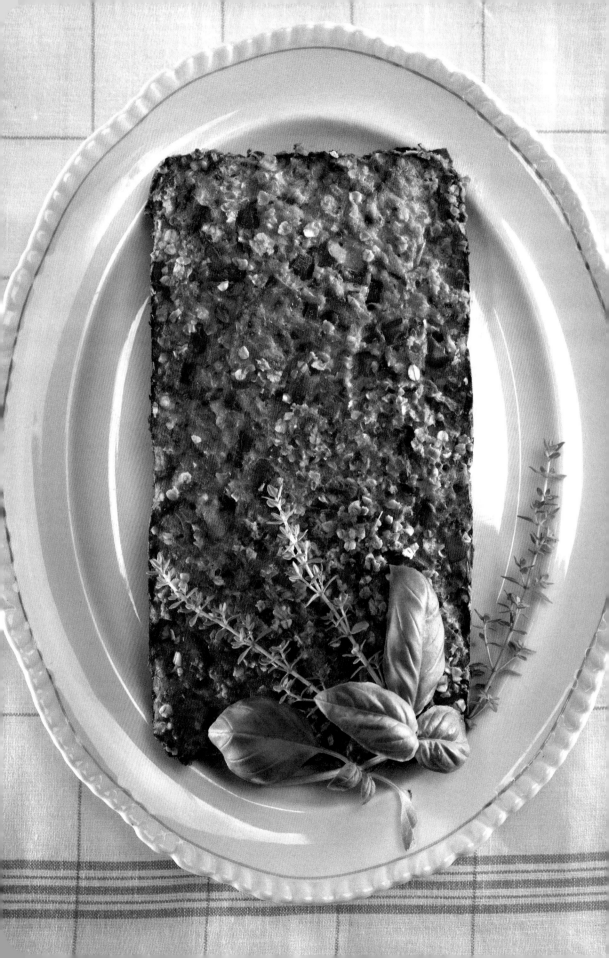

SALMON LOAF WITH VEGETABLES
AND HERBS

🍲 4 SERVINGS
10 MINUTES
35 MINUTES

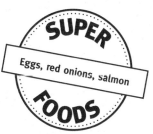

SUPER

Eggs, red onions, salmon

FOODS

INGREDIENTS

2 **eggs**, beaten

2 tbsp 2% milk

2 cans (each 6 oz/170 g) **salmon**, drained and flaked

½ cups (125 ml) rolled oats

1 carrot, grated

½ red or green pepper, finely diced

1 **red onion**, finely chopped

2 tbsp chopped fresh basil

Pinch dried oregano

Leaves of 1 sprig fresh thyme

Seasoning to taste

METHOD

Position rack in center of oven and preheat to 350°F (180°C).

In a medium bowl, combine all ingredients.

Oil an 8 x 4 inch (20 x 10 cm) bread tin. Pour mixture into tin and bake in center of preheated oven for about 35 minutes.

Let cool to room temperature before turning out.

COMMON MISCONCEPTIONS

Salmon is a fatty fish.

TRUE…but, while it is one of the fattiest fish, its percentage of fats is similar to that of lean meat. Plus, the fat in salmon is healthy fat.

Nutrition Facts Per serving	
Amount	**% Daily Value**
Calories 190	
Fat 8 g	12%
Saturated 2 g	
+ Trans 0 g	
Polyunsaturated 2.5 g	
Omega-6 1 g	
Omega-3 1 g	
Monounsaturated 3 g	
Cholesterol 105 mg	35%
Sodium 320 mg	14%
Potassium 450 mg	13%
Carbohydrates 15 g	5%
Fiber 3 g	12%
Sugar 4 g	
Protein 15 g	
Vitamin A 797 ER	80%
Vitamin C 24 mg	40%
Calcium 176 mg	15%
Iron 1.9 mg	15%
Phosphorus 744.2 mg	70%

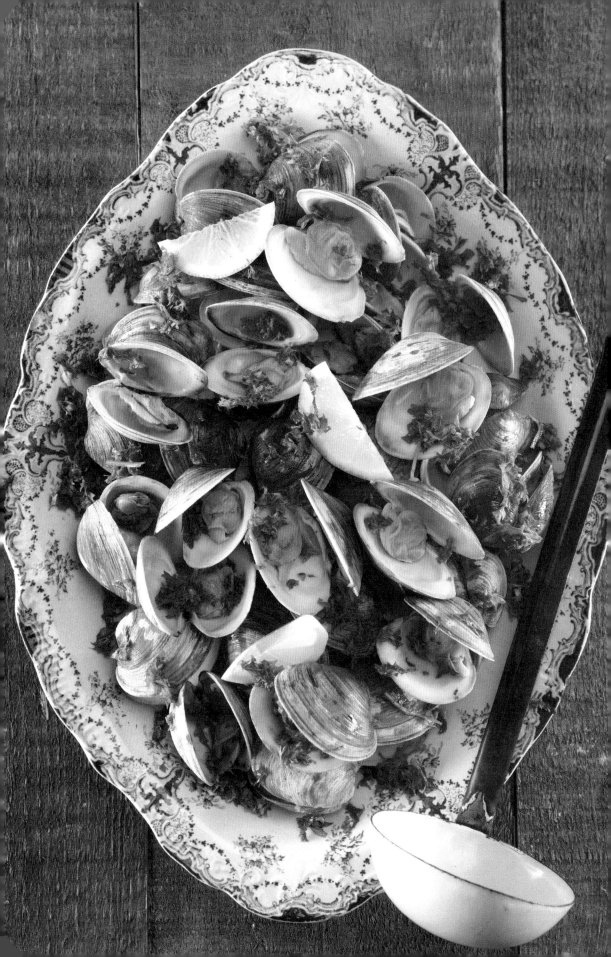

PORTUGUESE
CLAMS

4 SERVINGS
2 HOURS
40 MINUTES
15 MINUTES

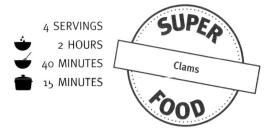

SUPER
Clams
FOOD

INGREDIENTS

48 small hard-shell **clams**

¼ cup (60 ml) olive oil

5 gloves garlic, finely chopped

1½ cups (375 ml) water

½ cup (125 ml) dry white wine

1 cup (250 ml) chopped fresh parsley

1 lemon, quartered

Seasoning to taste

METHOD

Wash clams. Let them soak in a large bowl of cold water for 2 hours, changing water two or three time. Rinse well and drain. (Do not pour contents of bowl in a strainer, or sand deposited at bottom will fall back onto clams.)

In a large saucepan, heat oil over medium-low heat and sauté garlic for 3 to 4 minutes. Add water and wine. Increase heat and bring to a boil.

Add clams, cover and cook for 3 to 5 minutes or until shells open. Garnish with parsley and season. Continue cooking, covered, for 5 minutes.

Serve with lemon quarters.

Nutrition Facts Per serving	
Amount	% Daily Value
Calories 210	
Fat 14 g	22%
Saturated 2 g	
+ Trans 0 g	
Polyunsaturated 1.5 g	
Omega-6 1.5 g	
Omega-3 0.3 g	
Monounsaturated 10 g	
Cholesterol 35 mg	12%
Sodium 70 mg	3%
Potassium 460 mg	13%
Carbohydrates 5 g	2%
Fiber 1 g	4%
Sugar 0 g	
Protein 15 g	
Vitamin A 224 ER	20%
Vitamin C 35 mg	60%
Calcium 80 mg	8%
Iron 1.63 mg	12%
Phosphorus 201.3 mg	20%

GRILLED SARDINES WITH
HONEY AND MINT

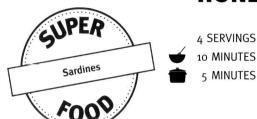

SUPER
Sardines
FOOD

4 SERVINGS

10 MINUTES

5 MINUTES

INGREDIENTS

2 tbsp olive oil

Juice of 1 lime or 1 lemon

1 tbsp honey

½ cup (125 ml) chopped fresh
mint leaves

1 tbsp ground cumin

2 cans (each 3.5 oz/100 g)
sardines in oil, drained

2 limes, quartered, for serving

Seasoning to taste

METHOD

In a bowl, combine oil, lime juice, honey, mint and cumin. Pour half of the marinade in another bowl.

Dip sardines in one bowl of marinade for a few seconds.

In a skillet over medium heat, grill sardines, turning partway through cooking, for 5 minutes.

Place sardines on plates. Pour unused marinade over sardines. Season and serve with lime quarters.

Nutrition Facts Per serving	
Amount	% Daily Value
Calories 200	
Fat 12 g	18%
Saturated 2.5 g	
+ Trans 0 g	
Polyunsaturated 2 g	
Omega-6 1 g	
Omega-3 1 g	
Monounsaturated 8 g	
Cholesterol 30 mg	10%
Sodium 210 mg	9%
Potassium 300 mg	9%
Carbohydrates 12 g	4%
Fiber 2 g	8%
Sugar 6 g	
Protein 11 g	
Vitamin A 63 ER	6%
Vitamin C 18 mg	30%
Calcium 168 mg	15%
Iron 3.6 mg	25%
Phosphorus 205.7 mg	20%

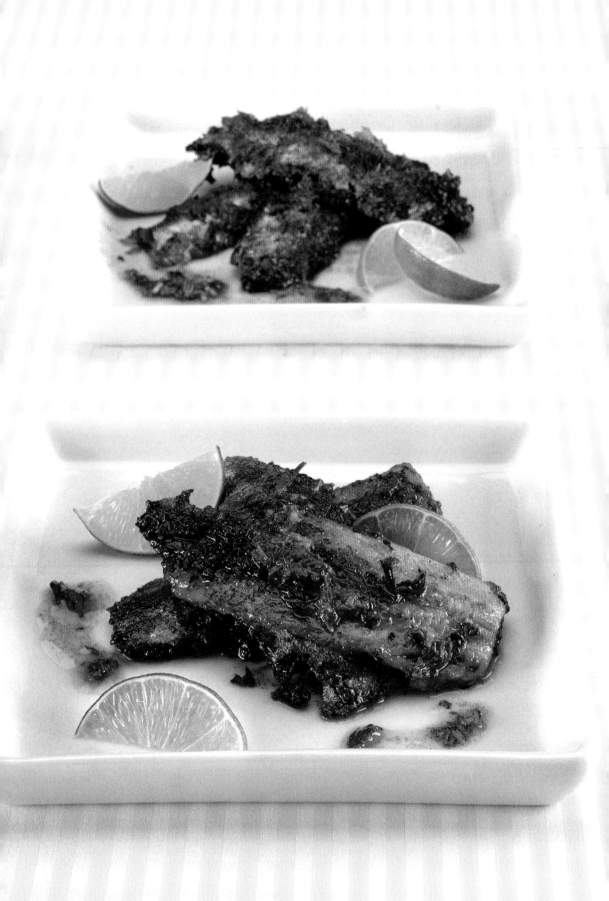

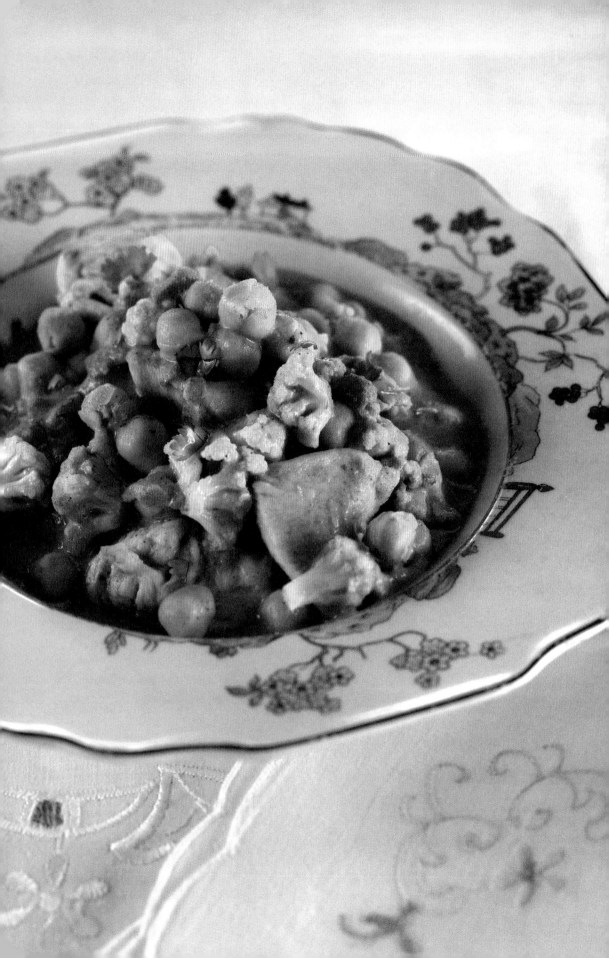

SPICY CHICKEN
WITH CHICKPEAS

6 SERVINGS
10 MINUTES
35 MINUTES

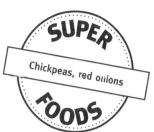

Chickpeas, red onions

INGREDIENTS

1 lb (454 g) boneless, skinless chicken breast, in pieces

Seasoning to taste

1 tbsp olive oil

1 large **red onion**, chopped

2 cloves garlic, finely chopped

1 tsp ground turmeric

1 tsp chopped fresh ginger

3 tbsp curry powder

1 cauliflower, in florets (about 6½ cups)

2 cans (each 14 oz/398 ml) diced tomatoes with no added salt

1 can (19 oz/540 ml) **chickpeas**, drained and rinsed

1 can (14 oz/398 ml) coconut milk

2 tbsp chopped fresh cilantro

METHOD

Season chicken.

In a large skillet, heat oil over medium-high heat and sauté onion and garlic for 2 minutes. Add chicken and cook for 3 to 5 minutes or until pieces start to brown. Reserve on a plate.

In a skillet over medium-high heat, add turmeric, ginger and curry. Cook for 2 minutes or until mixture is fragrant. Add cauliflower and tomatoes. Reduce heat to low. Cover and simmer for 8 to 10 minutes or until cauliflower is tender.

Return chicken to skillet and continue cooking, uncovered, stirring occasionally, for 10 to 15 minutes or until chicken pieces are cooked through, but still tender, and liquid thickens.

Add chickpeas and coconut milk. Remove from heat, season and garnish with cilantro.

Nutrition Facts Per serving		
Amount		% Daily Value
Calories 360		
Fat 8 g		12%
Saturated 1.5 g		
+ Trans 0 g		
Polyunsaturated 2 g		
Omega-6 1.5 g		
Omega-3 0.3 g		
Monounsaturated 3 g		
Cholesterol 60 mg		20%
Sodium 440 mg		18%
Potassium 1250 mg		36%
Carbohydrates 40 g		13%
Fiber 11 g		44%
Sugar 11 g		
Protein 33 g		
Vitamin A 52 ER		6%
Vitamin C 55 mg		90%
Calcium 157 mg		15%
Iron 5.5 mg		40%
Phosphorus 355 mg		30%

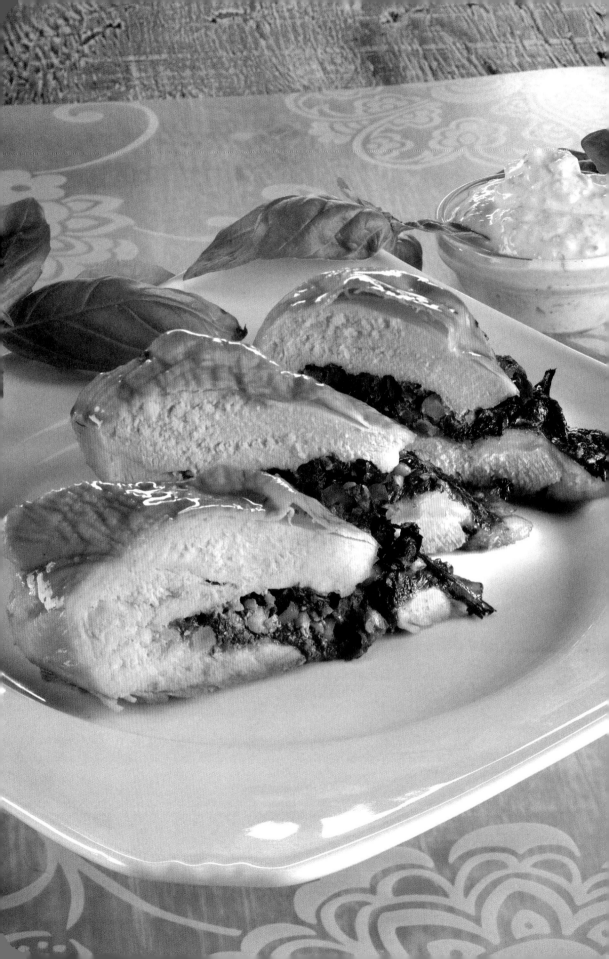

CHICKEN BREAST STUFFED WITH
BRIE AND SPINACH

4 SERVINGS
30 MINUTES
30 MINUTES

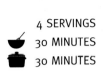

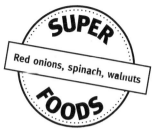
Red onions, spinach, walnuts

SUPER FOODS

INGREDIENTS

1 tbsp olive oil

1 small **red onion**, finely chopped

2 cloves garlic, finely chopped

2 cups (500 ml) baby **spinach**

2 boneless, skinless chicken breasts (1 lb/454 g)

3 oz (90 g) Brie (20% M.F. or less), without rind, sliced

2 tbsp chopped **walnuts**

2 tbsp chopped dried tomatoes

4 black olives, halved

For the sauce

⅔ cup (160 ml) plain Greek 0% M.F. yogurt

2 tbsp **Spinach** and **Walnut** Pesto (see recipe p. 90) or store-bought pesto

1 tsp maple syrup (optional)

Seasoning to taste

METHOD

Position rack in center of oven and preheat to 400°F (200°C).

In a skillet, heat oil over medium heat and sauté onion and garlic for 3 to 5 minutes. Add spinach and continue cooking for a few seconds. Transfer to a plate and sponge excess liquid with paper towel.

Slice chicken breast in two widthwise without completely cutting through it and open like a book.

Between each chicken breast half, place half of the cheese, spinach, walnuts, dried tomatoes and olives. Season and fold other half on top. Hold together with large toothpicks. Bake in center of preheated oven for 25 to 28 minutes.

Meanwhile, in a bowl, combine ingredients for sauce.

Cut stuffed chicken in half and top with sauce.

Nutrition Facts Per serving	
Amount	% Daily Value
Calories 380	
Fat 22 g	34%
Saturated 6 g + Trans 0.2 g	
Polyunsaturated 3.5 g	
Omega-6 3 g	
Omega-3 0.5 g	
Monounsaturated 9 g	
Cholesterol 95 mg	32%
Sodium 270 mg	11%
Potassium 460 mg	13%
Carbohydrates 7 g	2%
Fiber 1 g	4%
Sugar 4 g	
Protein 39 g	
Vitamin A 179 ER	20%
Vitamin C 7 mg	10%
Calcium 204 mg	20%
Iron 2.2 mg	15%
Phosphorus 330.4 mg	30%

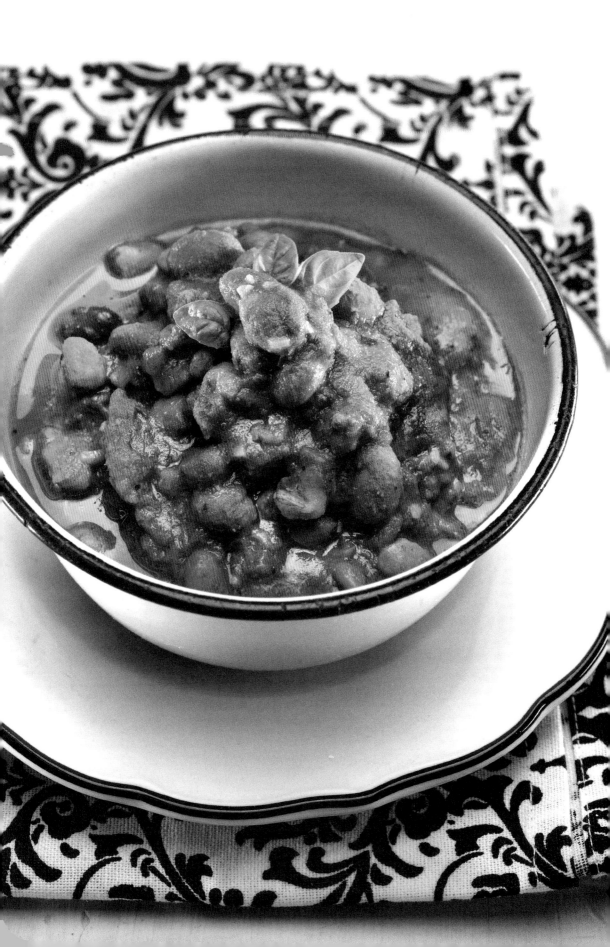

QUICK VEGETARIAN CHILI
WITH PINTO BEANS

🥣 4 SERVINGS
⬛ 20 MINUTES
🍲 15 MINUTES

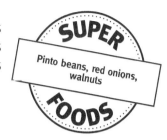

SUPER FOODS

Pinto beans, red onions, walnuts

INGREDIENTS

2 tbsp olive oil

1 **red onion**, chopped

4 cloves garlic, finely chopped

3 tbsp crushed **walnuts**

1 can (19 oz/540 ml) **pinto beans**, drained and rinsed

1 can (28 oz/796 ml) Italian tomatoes

1 tbsp dried oregano

1 tbsp ground turmeric

1 tbsp paprika

1 tsp dried basil

½ tsp dried thyme

2 pinches saffron (optional)

¼ tsp cayenne pepper

Seasoning to taste

METHOD

In a skillet, heat oil over medium heat and sauté onion, garlic and nuts for 3 to 5 minutes.

Add remaining ingredients and continue cooking, stirring often, for 10 minutes. Adjust seasoning.

PINTO BEANS AND FLATULENCE

Oligosaccharides (a sort of carbohydrate) are responsible for flatulence, large quantities of which are found in pinto beans. To eliminate as much as possible, it helps to give the beans a quick soak. This makes them faster to cook and easier to digest. To do this, place beans in a large saucepan of cold water. Bring to a boil over medium-high heat and then reduce heat and simmer for a minute or two. Remove the saucepan from the heat and let sit for 1 hour. Rinse beans under cold water before cooking. (The soaking water should be discarded.) For canned beans, just rinse thoroughly.

Nutrition Facts Per serving	
Amount	% Daily Value
Calories 280	
Fat 10 g	15%
Saturated 1.5 g	
+ Trans 0 g	
Polyunsaturated 3 g	
Omega-6 2.5 g	
Omega-3 0.5 g	
Monounsaturated 5 g	
Cholesterol 0 mg	0%
Sodium 800 mg	33%
Potassium 740 mg	21%
Carbohydrates 38 g	13%
Fiber 8 g	32%
Sugar 2 g	
Protein 10 g	
Vitamin A 179 ER	20%
Vitamin C 19 mg	30%
Calcium 147 mg	15%
Iron 4.7 mg	35%
Phosphorus 195.5 mg	20%

LENTIL AND
WALNUT BALLS

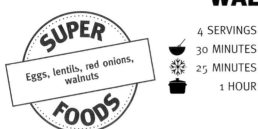

4 SERVINGS

30 MINUTES

25 MINUTES

1 HOUR

INGREDIENTS

4 cups (1 liter) water

1 cup (250 ml) dried green **lentils**

2 tbsp olive oil

1 **red onion**, chopped

2 cloves garlic, finely chopped

2 carrots, grated

2 cups (500 ml) chopped mushrooms

3 tbsp tomato paste

Leaves of 1 sprig fresh thyme

3 **eggs**, beaten

2 stalks celery, chopped

¼ cup (60 ml) chopped **walnuts**

½ cup (125 ml) grated Parmesan

½ cup (125 ml) chopped fresh parsley

¼ cup (60 ml) chopped fresh basil

¼ cup (60 ml) chia seeds or flaxseed

Seasoning to taste

METHOD

In a saucepan over high heat, bring water to a boil. Add lentils. Reduce heat to medium. Cover and simmer for 25 minutes or until tender, but not overcooked. Drain and let cool.

Meanwhile, in a skillet, heat oil over medium heat and sauté onion, garlic, carrots and mushrooms for 3 to 5 minutes. Add tomato paste, thyme and seasonings. Cook, stirring constantly, for about 3 minutes. Let cool.

In a large bowl, combine lentils, vegetables and remaining ingredients. Refrigerate for 25 minutes.

About 5 minutes before taking mixture out of refrigerator, position rack in center of oven and preheat to 400°F (200°C). Grease a baking sheet.

Shape 20 to 24 balls with your hands and place on prepared baking sheet. Bake in center of oven for about 3 minutes. Let balls cool for 5 minutes.

Serve with a sauce, if desired.

Nutrition Facts Per serving	
Amount	% Daily Value
Calories 520	
Fat 23 g	35%
Saturated 5 g	
+ Trans 0 g	
Polyunsaturated 8 g	
Omega-6 5 g	
Omega-3 3 g	
Monounsaturated 9 g	
Cholesterol 150 mg	50%
Sodium 320 mg	13%
Potassium 1140 mg	33%
Carbohydrates 49 g	16%
Fiber 14 g	56%
Sugar 9 g	
Protein 29 g	
Vitamin A 669 ER	70%
Vitamin C 27 mg	45%
Calcium 322 mg	30%
Iron 8 mg	60%
Phosphorus 584 mg	50%

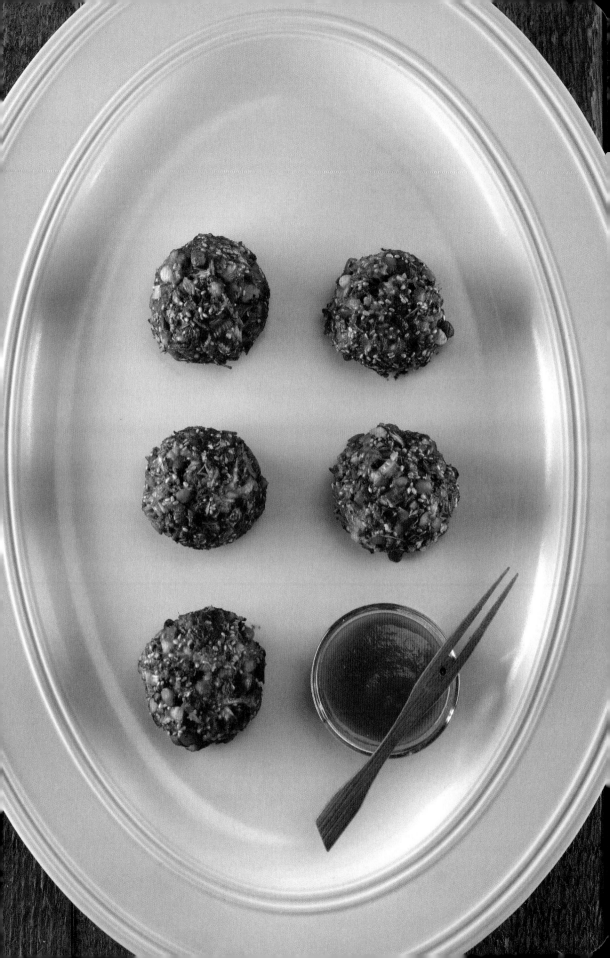

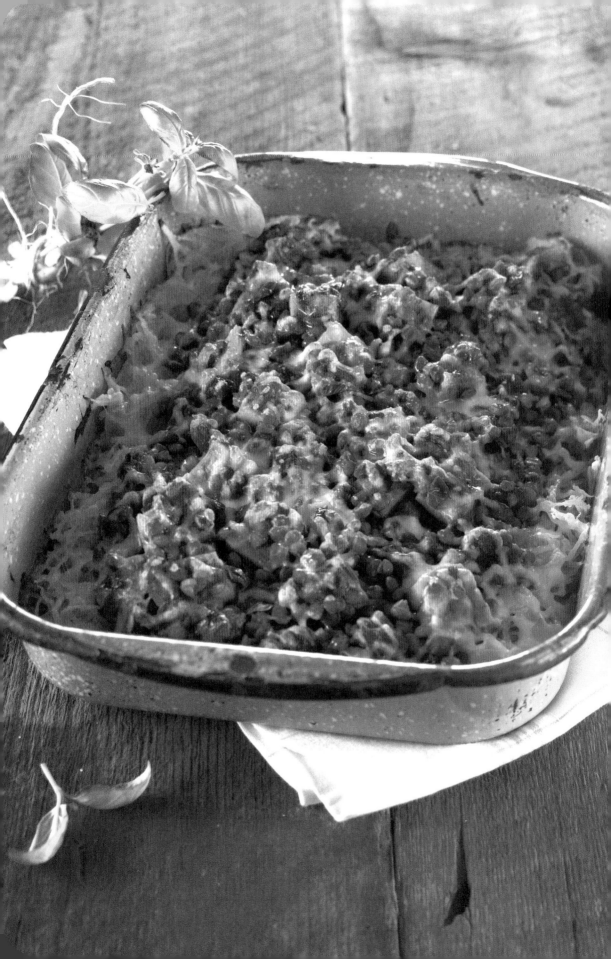

SPAGHETTI SQUASH WITH LENTILS
AND SWEET POTATO

4 SERVINGS
15 MINUTES
1 HOUR 20 MINUTES

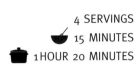

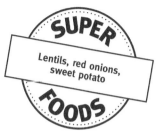

INGREDIENTS

2 spaghetti squash

1 tbsp olive oil

Seasoning to taste

½ cup (125 ml) grated mozzarella cheese

For the topping

2 tbsp olive oil

2 **red onions**, chopped

4 cloves garlic, finely chopped

1 **sweet potato**, diced

1 can (19 oz/540 ml) **lentils**, drained and rinsed

1 cup (250 ml) chicken or vegetable broth

2 tomatoes, diced

1 cup (250 ml) tomato sauce

½ cup (125 ml) finely chopped fresh basil

Leaves of 1 sprig fresh thyme

¼ tsp dried oregano

1 bay leaf

Seasoning to taste

METHOD

Position rack in center of oven and preheat to 375°F (190°C).

Cut squash in half lengthwise and remove seeds. On a baking sheet, place squash halves flesh side up. Brush with oil and season. Bake in center of preheated oven for 45 to 60 minutes or until tender. Let cool.

Meanwhile, in a skillet, heat oil over medium heat and sauté onions, garlic and sweet potato for 10 minutes. Add lentils, broth, tomatoes, tomato sauce and herbs. Continue cooking for 5 minutes.

Remove bay leaf and adjust seasoning.

In an ovenproof dish, separate squash into strands using a fork. Add topping and sprinkle with cheese.

Place under preheated oven broiler for 3 to 5 minutes or until cheese is golden.

Nutrition Facts Per serving		
Amount		**% Daily Value**
Calories 400		
Fat 16 g		25%
Saturated 3.5 g		
+ Trans 0.1 g		
Polyunsaturated 1.5 g		
Omega-6 1 g		
Omega-3 0.3 g		
Monounsaturated 7 g		
Cholesterol 10 mg		3%
Sodium 330 mg		14%
Potassium 890 mg		25%
Carbohydrates 49 g		16%
Fiber 9 g		36%
Sugar 14 g		
Protein 15 g		
Vitamin A 689 ER		70%
Vitamin C 24 mg		40%
Calcium 218 mg		20%
Iron 4.7 mg		35%
Phosphorus 218.7 mg	20%	

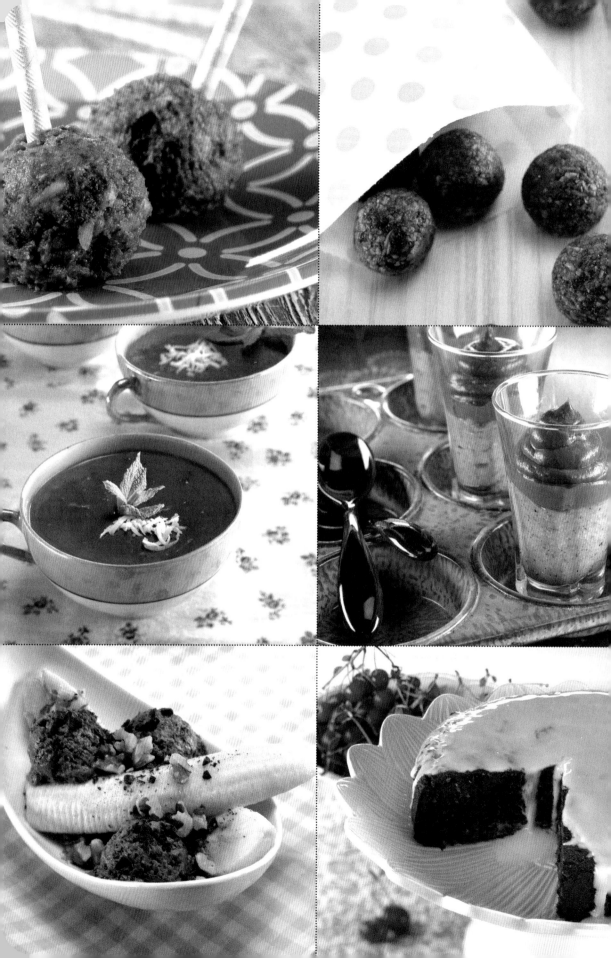

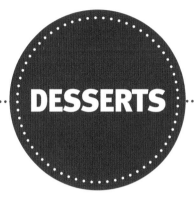

DESSERTS

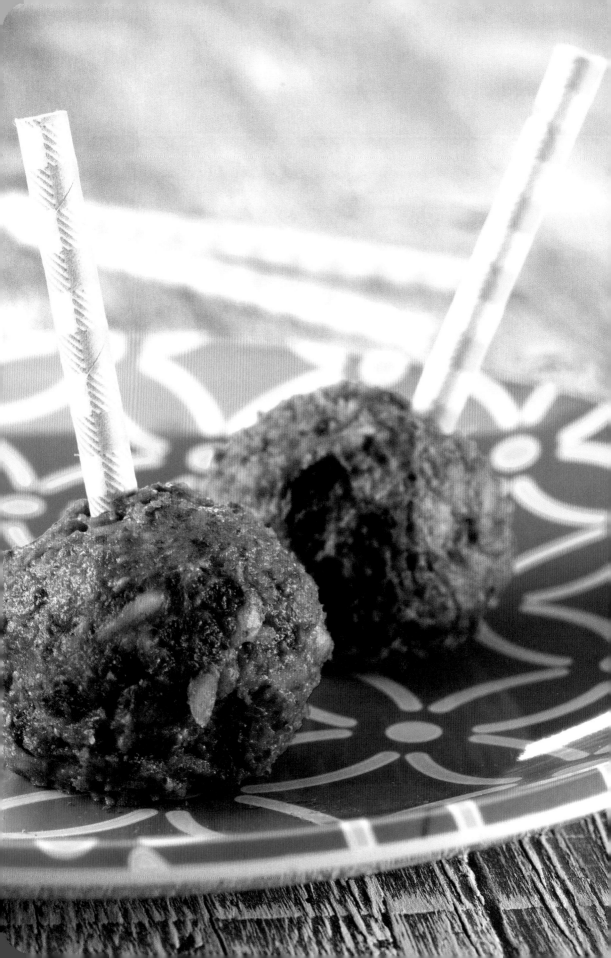

NUTRITIOUS
WALNUT BALLS

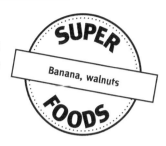

🥣 32 SERVINGS
15 MINUTES

SUPER FOODS

Banana, walnuts

INGREDIENTS

6 to 8 dried figs, chopped

¼ cup (60 ml) boiling water

2 cups (500 ml) **walnuts**

1 ripe **banana**, in pieces

1 cup (250 ml) chopped, pitted dates

METHOD

In a small bowl, cover figs with boiling water. Let sit for about 5 minutes to soften. Drain.

In a food processor, process nuts, banana, dates and figs to a smooth compote.

Shape 32 balls with your hands.

Refrigerate until ready to serve.

COMMON MISCONCEPTIONS

A banana is the equivalent of a steak.

FALSE. Bananas are as filling as meat, but, contrary to what many believe, they cannot replace a steak because they don't provide the same nutrients. The two foods are part of two separate food groups and their nutritional profiles are different. Bananas contain limited protein compared with steak, and they mainly provide carbohydrates, along with potassium and magnesium. However, a banana and a small steak have a similar number of calories.

Nutrition Facts Per serving		
Amount		**% Daily Value**
Calories 210		
Fat 5 g		8%
Saturated 0.5 g		
+ Trans 0 g		
Polyunsaturated 3.5 g		
Omega-6 3 g		
Omega-3 0.5 g		
Monounsaturated 0.5 g		
Cholesterol 0 mg		0%
Sodium 1 mg		0%
Potassium 380 mg		11%
Carbohydrates 40 g		13%
Fiber 5 g		20%
Sugar 32 g		
Protein 2 g		
Vitamin A 1 ER		0%
Vitamin C 1 mg		2%
Calcium 28 mg		2%
Iron 0.8 mg		6%
Phosphorus 58 mg		6%

SUNFLOWER SEED
TRUFFLES

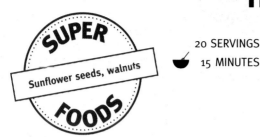

SUPER
Sunflower seeds, walnuts
FOODS

🥣 20 SERVINGS
15 MINUTES

INGREDIENTS

1 tbsp water

2 tbsp maple syrup

½ cup (125 ml) chopped pitted dates

1 cup (250 ml) **sunflower seeds**

½ cup (125 ml) **walnuts**

¼ cup (60 ml) grated, unsweetened coconut

¼ cup (60 ml) cocoa powder

METHOD

In a blender, add ingredients one by one. Blend for 1 minute or until a paste forms. Add water as needed.

Shape 20 small truffles by hand.

Refrigerate until ready to serve.

COMMON MISCONCEPTIONS

Chocolate is constipating.

FALSE. All varieties of chocolate contain fiber, which improves intestinal transit. Dark chocolate has twice the fiber of whole wheat bread or multigrain bread.

Nutrition Facts Per serving	
Amount	**% Daily Value**
Calories 100	
Fat 7 g	11%
Saturated 1.5 g	
+ Trans 0 g	
Polyunsaturated 4 g	
Omega-6 4 g	
Omega-3 0.3 g	
Monounsaturated 1 g	
Cholesterol 0 mg	0%
Sodium 1 mg	0%
Potassium 110 mg	3%
Carbohydrates 8 g	3%
Fiber 2 g	8%
Sugar 5 g	
Protein 2 g	
Vitamin A 0 ER	0%
Vitamin C 0 mg	0%
Calcium 12 mg	2%
Iron 0.8 mg	6%
Phosphorus 106.2 mg	10%

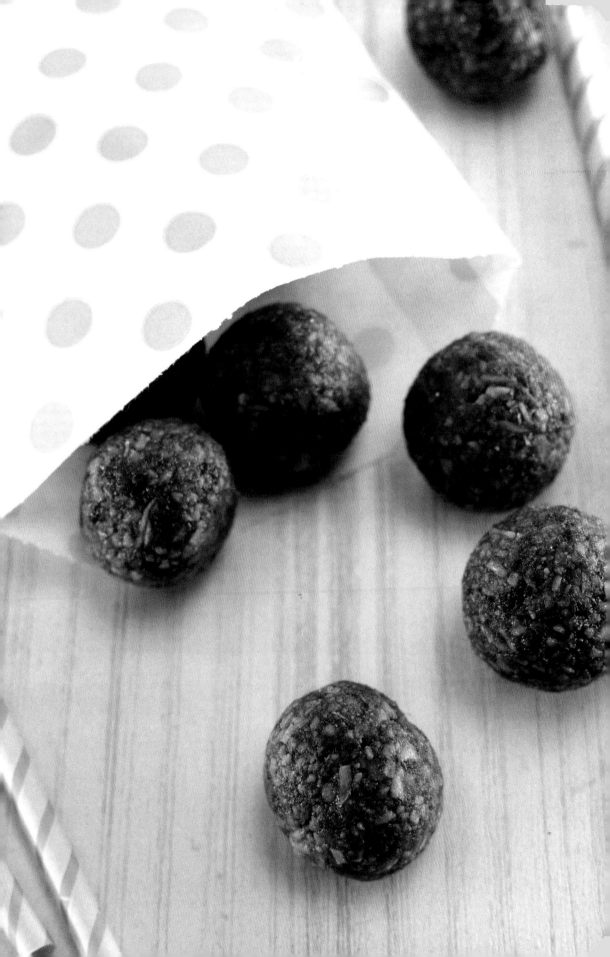

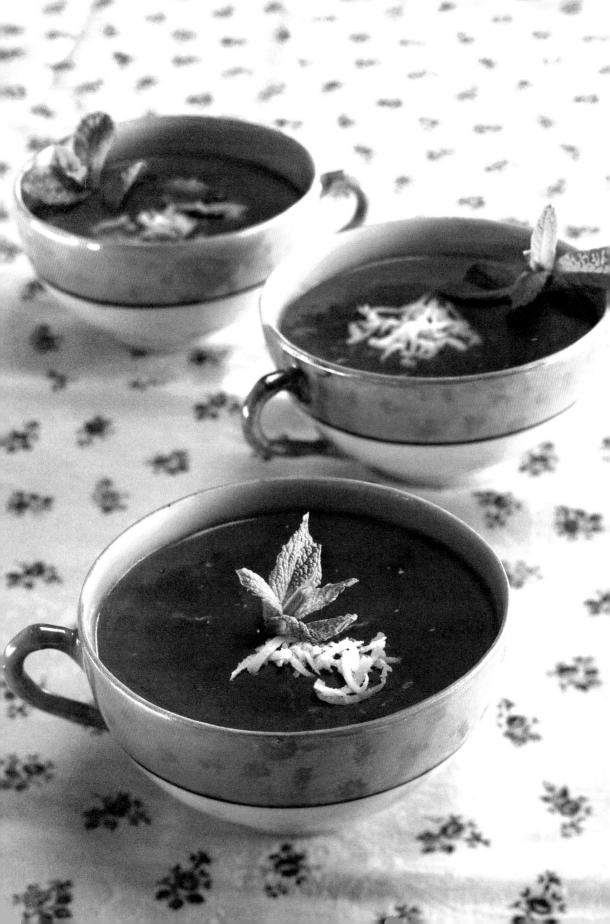

CHOCOLATY MINT
DESSERT

5 SERVINGS
15 MINUTES

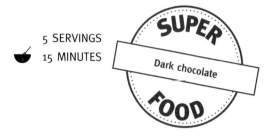

SUPER
Dark chocolate
FOOD

INGREDIENTS

3½ oz (100 g) **dark chocolate** (70% cocoa)

½ cup (125 ml) chopped pitted dates

½ can (14 oz/398 ml) coconut milk

1 tbsp chia seeds

2 tsp vanilla extract

1½ cups (375 ml) plain Greek yogurt

2 tbsp grated, unsweetened coconut

5 fresh mint leaves

METHOD

In a bain-marie, melt chocolate and add dates, coconut milk, chia seeds and vanilla. Gradually incorporate yogurt, adjusting quantity for desired consistency.

Distribute into dessert cups and garnish with coconut and mint leaves. Refrigerate.

COMMON MISCONCEPTIONS
Chocolate is fattening.
FALSE...but, as with any fatty, sweet food, it can contribute to weight gain if eaten regularly in large quantities. Studies show that regular eaters of dark chocolate are no more often overweight than non-eaters. Eat a small square of chocolate at the end of a meal rather than in the middle of the day to avoid sugar spikes, which promote weight gain.

Nutrition Facts Per serving	
Amount	**% Daily Value**
Calories 200	
Fat 7 g	11%
Saturated 4 g	
+ Trans 0 g	
Polyunsaturated 0.4 g	
Omega-6 0.1 g	
Omega-3 0.3 g	
Monounsaturated 0.1 g	
Cholesterol 1 mg	0%
Sodium 85 mg	4%
Potassium 200 mg	6%
Carbohydrates 26 g	9%
Fiber 4 g	16%
Sugar 20 g	
Protein 9 g	
Vitamin A 7 ER	0%
Vitamin C 1 mg	2%
Calcium 89 mg	8%
Iron 1.1 mg	8%
Phosphorus 33 mg	4%

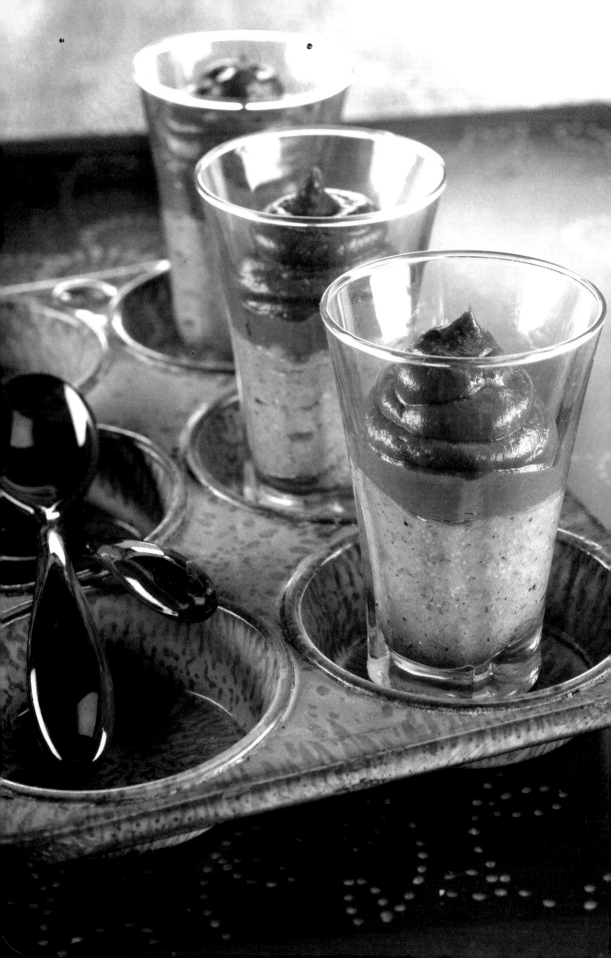

NUT-CRUSTED
DESSERT

8 SERVINGS
15 MINUTES
1 HOUR

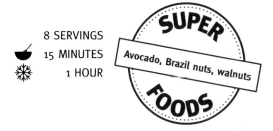

SUPER FOODS

Avocado, Brazil nuts, walnuts

INGREDIENTS

For the crust

3 tbsp coconut oil

½ cup (125 ml) cashews

¼ cup (60 ml) **Brazil nuts**

¼ cup (60 ml) **walnuts**

1 tsp maple syrup

½ tsp vanilla extract

For the cream

1 ripe **avocado**

2 tbsp maple syrup

1 tbsp honey

1 tbsp cocoa powder

1 tsp vanilla extract

METHOD

In a blender, blend ingredients for crust until they form a paste. Press mixture into bottom of 8 verrines. Refrigerate for 1 hour.

Meanwhile, in a blender, blend ingredients for cream until smooth and creamy. Add a bit of water as needed.

Top verrines with cream. Serve immediately.

Nutrition Facts Per serving	
Amount	% Daily Value
Calories 230	
Fat 19 g	29%
Saturated 7 g + Trans 0 g	
Polyunsaturated 4 g	
Omega-6 3.5 g	
Omega-3 0.4 g	
Monounsaturated 6 g	
Cholesterol 0 mg	0%
Sodium 3 mg	0%
Potassium 260 mg	7%
Carbohydrates 11 g	4%
Fiber 3 g	12%
Sugar 5 g	
Protein 4 g	
Vitamin A 5 ER	0%
Vitamin C 7 mg	10%
Calcium 24 mg	2%
Iron 1 mg	8%
Phosphorus 112 mg	10%

BANANA
SPLIT

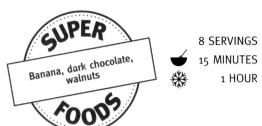

8 SERVINGS

15 MINUTES

1 HOUR

INGREDIENTS

4 ripe **bananas**, split in two lengthwise

4 oz (120 g) **dark chocolate** (80% cocoa)

¼ cup (60 ml) crushed **walnuts**

For the frozen yogurt

1 cup (250 ml) plain Greek yogurt

2 cups (500 ml) fresh blueberries or raspberries

2 tbsp honey or maple syrup

METHOD

In a food processor, process ingredients for frozen yogurt and freeze for 1 hour at most. If you leave yogurt in longer, it will be too hard.

In long dishes, place bananas and top with scoops of frozen yogurt.

Grate chocolate and melt in a bain-marie.

Top bananas with chocolate and nuts.

Put 2 portions on a plate and share with someone!

Nutrition Facts Per serving	
Amount	**% Daily Value**
Calories 230	
Fat 8 g	12%
Saturated 3.5 g + Trans 0 g	
Polyunsaturated 2 g	
Omega-6 1.5 g	
Omega-3 0.4 g	
Monounsaturated 0.4 g	
Cholesterol 0 mg	0%
Sodium 30 mg	1%
Potassium 250 mg	7%
Carbohydrates 33 g	11%
Fiber 3 g	12%
Sugar 23 g	
Protein 6 g	
Vitamin A 6 ER	0%
Vitamin C 9 mg	15%
Calcium 40 mg	4%
Iron 0.8 mg	6%
Phosphorus 30 mg	2%

—— DID YOU KNOW? ——

White chocolate is made from cocoa butter and not cocoa powder; it contains only sugar and fat.

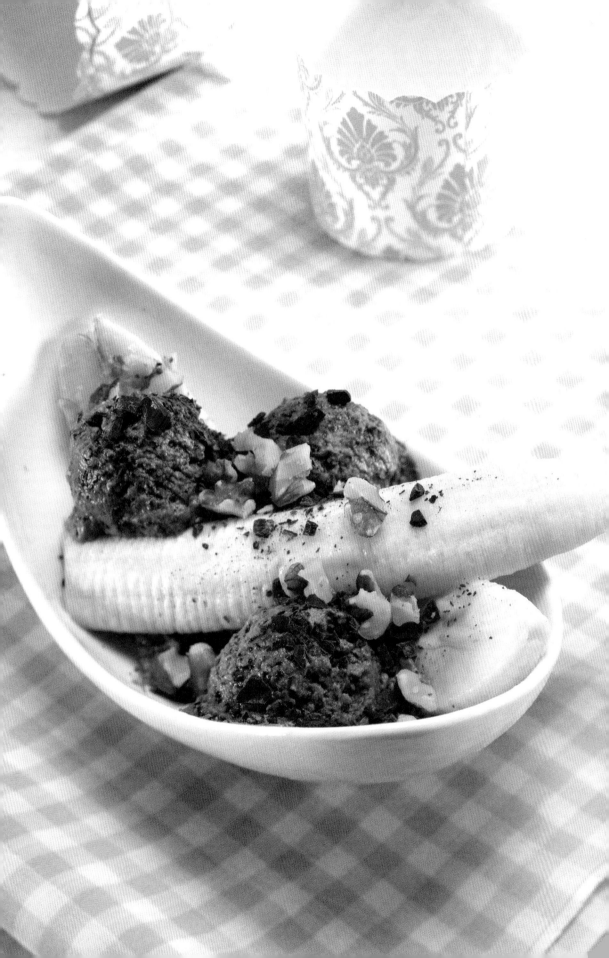

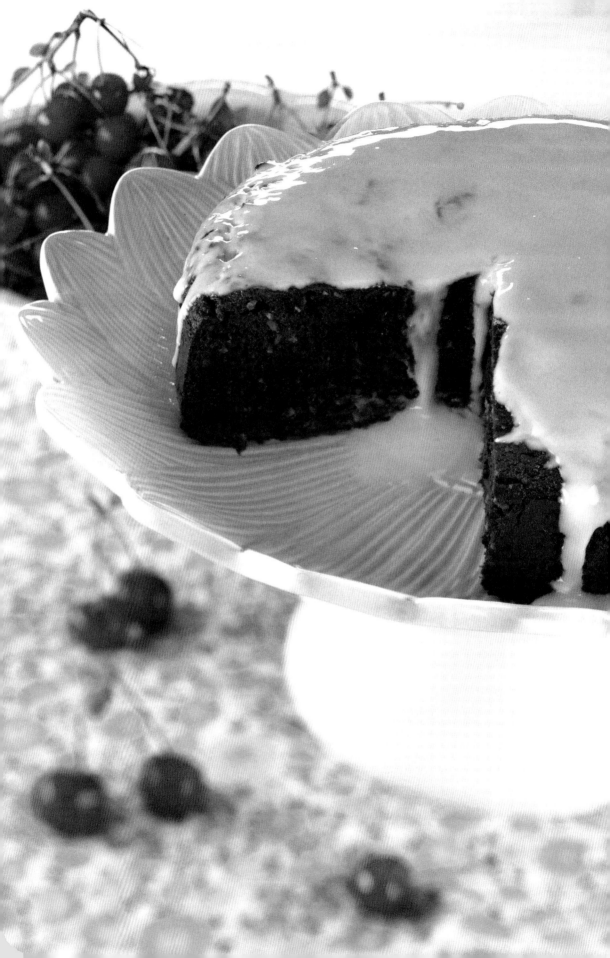

FLOURLESS CHOCOLATE
HAZELNUT CAKE

16 SERVINGS
20 MINUTES
40 MINUTES

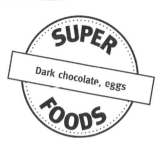

SUPER FOODS

Dark chocolate, eggs

INGREDIENTS

6 **eggs**

2½ cups (625 ml) hazelnuts, ground

½ cup (125 ml) date purée

½ cup (125 ml) cocoa powder

¼ cup (60 ml) olive oil or coconut oil

½ cup (125 ml) unsweetened applesauce

1 tsp baking powder

1 tsp baking soda

¼ cup (60 ml) **dark chocolate** chips

For the icing

½ cup (125 ml) plain yogurt

¼ cup (60 ml) honey or maple syrup

METHOD

Position rack in center of oven and preheat to 350°F (180°C). Grease 9-inch (23 cm) round cake tin.

Separate egg yolks and whites. Place whites in a large bowl and yolks in a blender.

Using an electric mixer, beat egg whites until stiff peaks form. Reserve.

In blender, blend hazelnuts and egg yolks. Then add date purée, cocoa, oil, applesauce, baking powder and baking soda. Blend again.

Gently combine mixture with egg whites. Add chocolate chips and blend.

Pour mixture into prepared cake tin and bake in center of oven for about 40 minutes. Let cool and turn out.

Meanwhile, combine yogurt and honey in a bowl and spread icing over cake.

COMMON MISCONCEPTIONS

Dark chocolate has fewer calories than milk chocolate.

FALSE. All chocolate has approximately the same number of calories. Paradoxically, 89% dark chocolate has more fat and less sugar than milk chocolate. But dark chocolate offers more nutritional benefits than other chocolate.

Nutrition Facts Per serving	
Amount	**% Daily Value**
Calories 200	
Fat 12 g	18%
Saturated 2.5 g	
+ Trans 0 g	
Polyunsaturated 1 g	
Omega-6 1 g	
Omega-3 0.1 g	
Monounsaturated 8 g	
Cholesterol 70 mg	23%
Sodium 150 mg	6%
Potassium 160 mg	5%
Carbohydrates 19 g	6%
Fiber 2 g	8%
Sugar 16 g	
Protein 5 g	
Vitamin A 29 ER	2%
Vitamin C 1 mg	2%
Calcium 68 mg	6%
Iron 1.2 mg	8%
Phosphorus 94 mg	8%

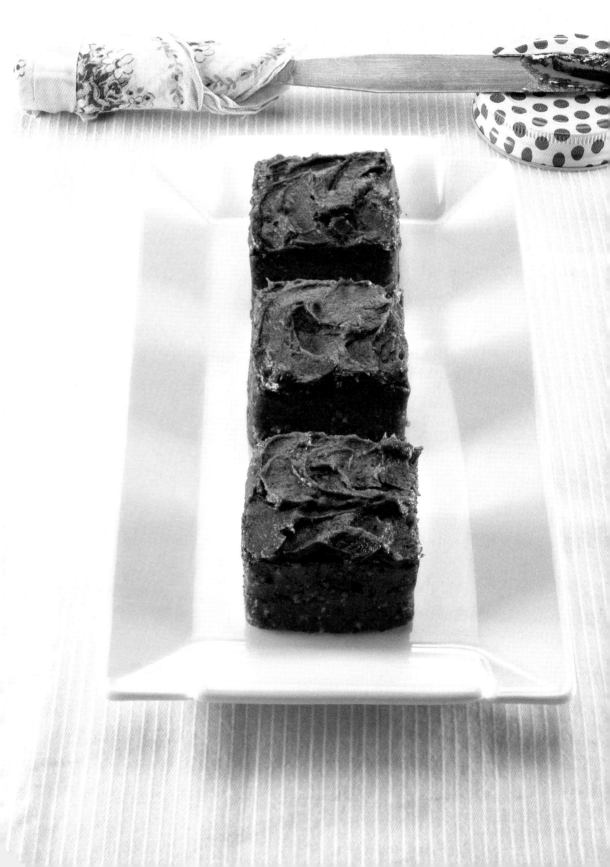

BAKELESS
BANANA NUT CAKE

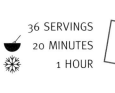

36 SERVINGS
20 MINUTES
1 HOUR

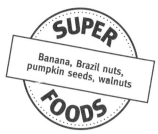

Banana, Brazil nuts, pumpkin seeds, walnuts

INGREDIENTS

For the crust

1 tbsp water

1½ cups (375 ml) chopped pitted dates

1 cup (250 ml) **Brazil nuts**

1 cup (250 ml) **walnuts**

½ cup (125 ml) **pumpkin seeds**

For the filling

¼ cup (60 ml) water

3 tbsp maple syrup

3 tbsp coconut oil

2 tbsp cocoa powder

2 cups (500 ml) cashews

1 **banana**, in pieces

For the ganache

½ cup (125 ml) coconut oil

2 tbsp maple syrup

2 tbsp cocoa powder

METHOD

In a blender, blend ingredients for crust into small pieces. Add water as needed, so mixture sticks together when pressed with fingers.

Spread mixture in bottom of 9 x 9 inch (23 x 23 cm) tin. Press with fingers and refrigerate.

In a blender, blend ingredients for filling until smooth. Add water as needed. Pour mixture over crust and refrigerate for 1 hour.

Meanwhile, in a small bowl, whisk together ingredients for ganache.

Turn cake out and spread ganache on filling with a spatula. Refrigerate until ready to serve.

Nutrition Facts Per serving	
Amount	**% Daily Value**
Calories 190	
Fat 14 g	22%
Saturated 6 g	
+ Trans 0 g	
Polyunsaturated 3.5 g	
Omega-6 3 g	
Omega-3 0.3 g	
Monounsaturated 4 g	
Cholesterol 0 mg	0%
Sodium 2 mg	0%
Potassium 180 mg	5%
Carbohydrates 13 g	4%
Fiber 2 g	8%
Sugar 8 g	
Protein 3 g	
Vitamin A 1 ER	0%
Vitamin C 0 mg	0%
Calcium 20 mg	2%
Iron 1.2 mg	8%
Phosphorus 112 mg	10%

BAKELESS
BRAZIL NUT CAKE

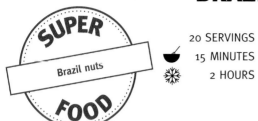

20 SERVINGS

15 MINUTES

2 HOURS

INGREDIENTS

3 cups (750 ml) **Brazil nuts**

3 cups (750 ml) almonds

3 tbsp cocoa powder

1 cup (250 ml) chopped pitted dates

¼ cup (60 ml) freshly squeezed orange juice

2 tbsp coconut oil

A few **Brazil nuts**, coarsely chopped, for decoration

METHOD

In a food processor, process Brazil nuts, almonds and cocoa.

Add dates, orange juice and oil. Process for 30 to 60 seconds or until mixture forms a paste.

Pour mixture in a 9-inch (23 cm) round cake tin and refrigerate for 2 hours.

Decorate with chopped Brazil nuts.

COMMON MISCONCEPTIONS

Chocolate causes migraines.

FALSE...but it can provoke headaches in people who suffer from them because of its content of theobromine. But no scientific studies have pointed to chocolate as causing migraines. Science has proven the opposite by giving chocolate to patients who suffer from migraines via a feeding tube in the stomach, without them knowing what they were being given: no migraines were observed.

Nutrition Facts Per serving	
Amount	**% Daily Value**
Calories 360	
Fat 29 g	45%
Saturated 6 g	
+ Trans 0 g	
Polyunsaturated 8 g	
Omega-6 8 g	
Omega-3 0 g	
Monounsaturated 13 g	
Cholesterol 0 mg	0%
Sodium 5 mg	0%
Potassium 390 mg	11%
Carbohydrates 15 g	5%
Fiber 5 g	20%
Sugar 8 g	
Protein 9 g	
Vitamin A 1 ER	0%
Vitamin C 2 mg	2%
Calcium 90 mg	8%
Iron 1.6 mg	10%
Phosphorus 294.5 mg	25%

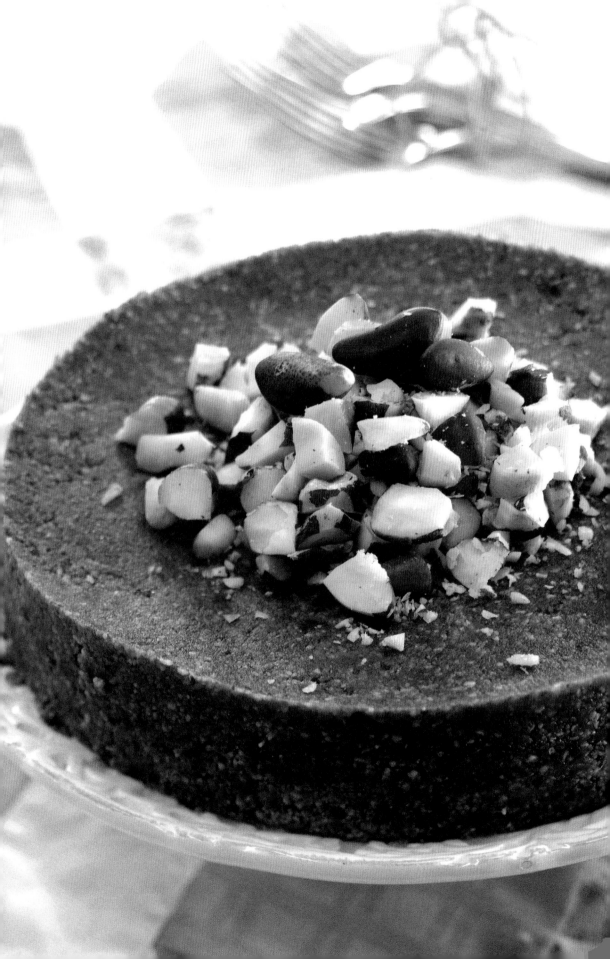

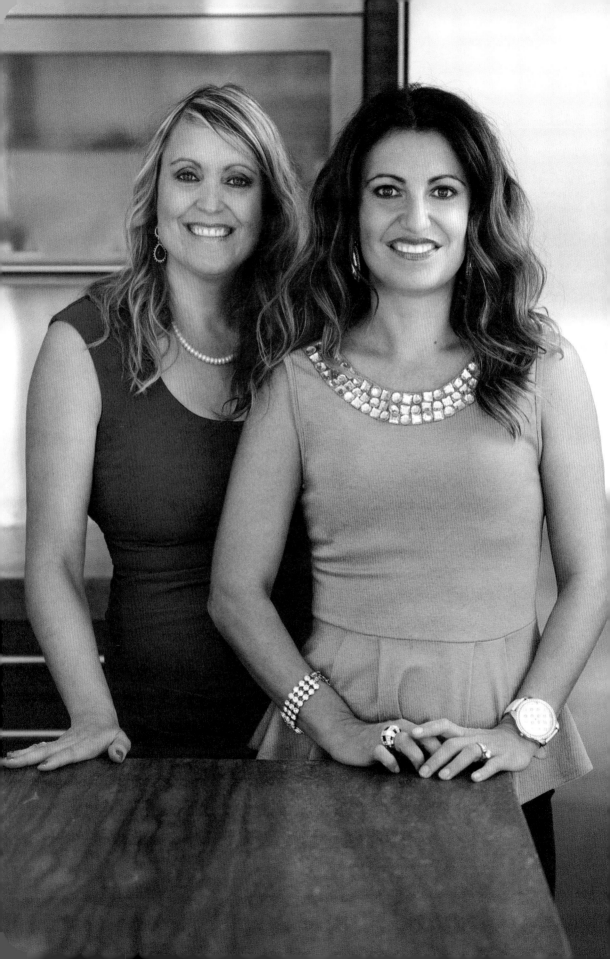

ACKNOWLEDGMENTS

Thank you to Marc G. Alain and Isabelle Jodoin at Modus Vivendi Publishing for giving us the chance to be part of the new Superfoods series. Thanks to Nolwenn Gouezel, who offered invaluable assistance researching and writing this book. Thanks also to Émilie Houle, graphic designer.

Thanks to photographer André Noël and food stylist Gabrielle Dalessandro for making our recipes even more appetizing, as well as Camille Gyrya for our photos and other pictures.

Thank you to our science committee for verifying the information.

Thanks to our chef, Michael Linnington, who added his delicate touch to our recipes.

And thanks to the loves of our lives: our spouses, Jack and Pierre, who patiently supported us while we wrote this book, and our children, Eza, Oceana, Xavier and Jessica, Dominique and Valérie, who drive us to follow our dreams.

We hope with all our hearts that you achieve your life's goals.

Thank you to everyone who buys this book or consults us at a clinic. Be sure to visit our website (nutrisimple.com).

Marise Charron and Elisabeth Cerqueira
nutrisimple.com

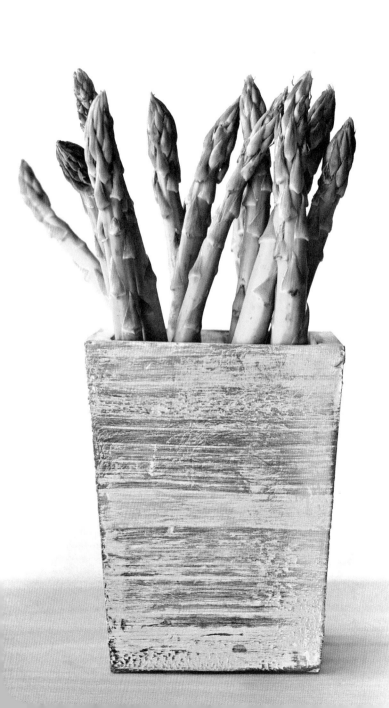

SCIENTIFIC
REFERENCES

Anglin, R. E., Z. Samaan, S. D. Walter, and S. D. McDonald. "Vitamin D deficiency and depression in adults: systematic review and meta-analysis." *The British Journal of Psychiatry* 202, no. 2 (2013): 100–107.

Asselin, P. "Carence en vitamine B_{12}: conséquences graves à appréhender." Chronique Santé, *Le soleil*, May 9, 2009. http://www.lapresse.ca/le-soleil/actualites/sante/200905/08/01-854874-carence-en-vitamine-b12-consequences-graves-a-apprehender.php.

Benton, D. "Selenium intake, mood and other aspects of psychological functioning." *Nutritional Neuroscience* 5, no. 6 (2002): 363–74.

Carlezon, W. A., Jr., S. D. Mague, A. M. Parow, A. L. Stoll, B. M. Cohen, and P. F. Renshaw. "Antidepressant-like effects of uridine and omega-3 fatty acids are potentiated by combined treatment in rats." *Biological Psychiatry* 57, no. 4 (2005): 343–50.

Collectif. "Tout sur les fruits, les noix et les graines." In *L'Encyclopédie des aliments*, Vol. 2. Montreal: Québec Amérique, 2014.

Collectif. "Tout sur les légumes." In *L'Encyclopédie des aliments*, Vol. 1. Montreal: Québec Amérique, 2013.

Coppen, A., and J. Bailey. "Enhancement of the antidepressant action of fluoxetine by folic acid: a randomized placebo controlled trial." *Journal of Affective Disorders* 60 (2000): 121–30.

Curtay, J. P. "Le manque de magnésium peut-il avoir une influence sur la dépression?" Accessed June 2014. http://www.allodocteurs.fr/actualite-sante-le-manque-de-magnesium-peut-il-avoir-une-influence-sur-la-depression-_13079.html.

Duffield, A. J., and C. D. Thomson. "A comparison of methods of assessment of dietary intakes in Otago, New Zealand." *British Journal of Nutrition* 82, no. 2 (1999): 131–38.

Fava, M., J. S. Borus, J. E. Alpert, A. A. Nierenberg, J. F. Rosenbaum, and T. Bottiglieri. "Folate, vitamin B_{12}, and homocysteine in major depressive disorder." *The American Journal of Psychiatry* 154, no. 3 (1997): 426–28.

Grosso, G., F. Galvano, S. Marventano, M. Malaguarnera, C. Bucolo, F. Drago, and F. Caraci. "Omega-3 fatty acids and depression: scientific evidence and biological mechanisms." *Oxidative Medicine and Cellular Longevity* 2014 (2014): Article 313570.

Hibbeln, J. R. "Seafood consumption, the DHA content of mothers' milk and prevalence rates of postpartum depression: a cross-national, ecological analysis." *Journal of Affective Disorders* 69, no. 1–3 (2002): 15–29.

Hurley, L. L., L. Akinfiresoye, O. Kalejayle, and Y. Tizabi. "Antidepressant effects of resveratrol in an animal model of depression." *Behavioural Brain Research* 268 (2014): 1–7.

Jacka, F. N., J. A. Pasco, M. J. Henry, M. A. Kotowicz, G. C. Nicholson, and M. Berk. "Dietary omega-3 fatty acids and depression in a community sample." *Nutritional Neuroscience* 7, no. 2 (2004): 101–6.

Lespérance, F., N. Frasure-Smith, E. St-André, G. Turecki, P. Lespérance, and S. R. Wisniewski. "The efficacy of omega-3 supplementation for major depression: a randomized controlled trial." *The Journal of Clinical Psychiatry* 72, no. 8 (2011): 1054–62.

Liu, D., K. Xie, X. Yang et al. "Resveratrol reverses the effects of chronic unpredictable mild stress on behavior, serum corticosterone levels and BDNF expression in rats." *Behavioural Brain Research* 264 (2014): 9–16.

Mamalakis, G., M. Tornaritis, and A. Kafatos. "Depression and adipose essential polyunsaturated fatty acids." *Prostaglandins, Leukotrienes and Essential Fatty Acids* 67, no. 5 (2002): 311–18.

Martin, F. P. J., S. Rezzi, E. Peré-Trepat et al. "Metabolic effects of dark chocolate consumption on energy, gut microbiota, and stress-related metabolism in free-living subjects." *Journal of Proteome Research* 8, no. 12 (2009): 5568–79.

Morris, D. W., M. H. Trivedi, and A. J. Rush. "Folate and unipolar depression." *The Journal of Alternative and Complementary Medicine* 14, no. 3 (2008): 277–85.

Nutra News. "Combattre la dépression par des suppléments nutritionnels naturels." Accessed June 2014. http://www.nutranews.org/sujet.pl?id=223.

Nutri-Facts. "Acides gras essentiels: dépression majeure et trouble bipolaire." Accessed June 2014. http://www.nutri-facts.org/fra/acides-gras-essentiels/acides-gras-essentiels/autres-applications/.

Nutri-Facts. "Micronutriments et dépression." Theme for February 2012. Accessed June 2014. http://archive.nutri-facts.org/fra/theme-du-mois/detail/backPid/94/article/micronutriments-et-depression/.

Passeportsanté.net. "Diète spéciale: dépression." Accessed June 2014. http://www.passeportsante.net/fr/Nutrition/Dietes/Fiche.aspx?doc=diete-depression.

Pathak, L., Y. Agrawal, and A. Dhir. "Natural polyphenols in the management of major depression." *Expert Opinion on Investigational Drugs* 22, no. 7 (2013): 863–80.

Quirk, S. E., L. J. Williams, A. O'Neil et al. "The association between diet quality, dietary patterns and depression in adults: a systematic review." *BMC Psychiatry* 13, no. 1 (2013): 175–97.

Ravindran, A. V., R. W. Lam, M. J. Filteau, F. Lespérance, S. H. Kennedy, S. V. Parikh, and S. B. Patten. Canadian Network for Mood and Anxiety Treatments (CANMAT). "Clinical guidelines for the management of major depressive disorder in adults. V. Complementary and alternative medicine treatments." *Journal of Affective Disorders* 117, suppl. 1 (2009): S54–S64.

Sánchez-Villegas, A., M. A. Martínez-González, R. Estruch et al. "Mediterranean dietary pattern and depression: the PREDIMED randomized trial." *BMC Medicine* 11 (2013): 208–19.

Schueller, G. H. "Winter depression? Eat these foods to help treat seasonal affective disorder (SAD)." *Eating Well* online. Page accessed June 2014. http://www.eatingwell.com/nutrition_health/nutrition_news_information/winter_depression_eat_these_foods_to_help_treat_seasonal_affective_disorder_sad.

Seppälä, J., A. Kauppinen, H. Kautiainen, M. Vanhala, and H. Koponen. "Depression and diet." *Duodecim* 130, no. 9 (2014): 902–9.

Skarupski, K. A., C. Tangney, H. Li, B. Ouyang, D. A. Evans, and M. C. Morris. "Longitudinal association of vitamin B_6, folate, and vitamin B_{12} with depressive symptoms among older adults over time." *The American Journal of Clinical Nutrition* 92, no. 2 (2010): 330–35.

Stein, T. "Depression won't go away? Folate could be the answer." *Psychology Today* online. Accessed June 2014. http://www.psychologytoday.com/blog/the-integrationist/201310/depression-wont-go-away-folate-could-be-the-answer.

Stranges, S., P. C. Samaraweera, F. Taggart, N. B. Kandala, and S. Stewart-Brown. "Major health-related behaviours and mental well-being in the general population: the Health Survey for England." *BMJ Open* 4, no. 9 (2014): e005878.

Su, K. P., S. Y. Huang, C. C. Chiu, and W. W. Shen. "Omega-3 fatty acids in major depressive disorder: a preliminary double-blind, placebo-controlled trial." *European Neuropsychopharmacology* 13, no. 4 (2003): 267–71.

Swardfager, W., N. Hermann, G. Mazereeuw, K. Goldberger, T. Harimoto, and K. L. Lanctôt. "Zinc in depression: a meta-analysis." *Biological Psychiatry* 74, no. 12 (2013): 872–78.

Taylor, M. J., S. M. Carney, G. M. Goodwin, and J. R. Geddes. "Folate for depressive disorders: systematic review and meta-analysis of randomized controlled trials." *Journal of Psychopharmacology* 18, no. 2 (2004): 251–56.

Thomson, C. D., A. Chisholm, S. K. McLachlan, and J. M. Campbell. "Brazil nuts: an effective way to improve selenium status." *The American Journal of Clinical Nutrition* 87, no. 2 (2008): 379–84.

Tolmunen, T., J. Hintikka, A. Ruusunen et al. "Dietary folate and the risk of depression in Finnish middle-aged men: a prospective follow-up study." *Psychotherapy and Psychosomatics* 73, no. 6 (2004): 334–39.

Young, S. N. "Folate and depression: a neglected problem." *Journal of Psychiatry & Neuroscience* 32, no. 2 (2007): 80–82.

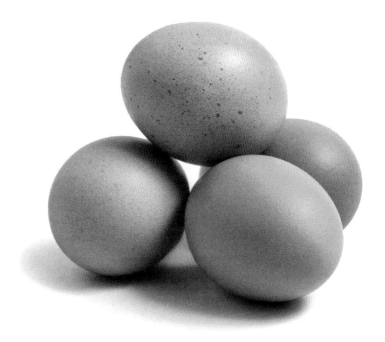

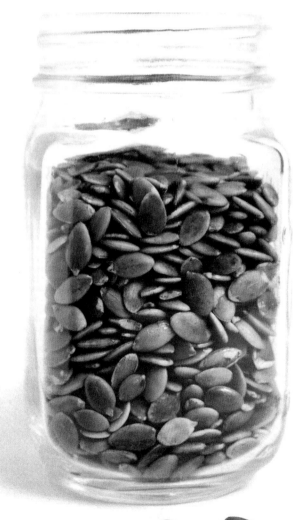
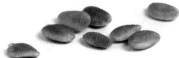

GLOSSARY

AMINO ACIDS
Elements that make up proteins. The body needs 20 amino acids to grow and function, but it produces only 11 of them. The nine others are called essential, because the human body cannot produce them so they have to come exclusively from diet. *See* Protein.

ANTIOXIDANTS
Compounds that help prevent oxidative stress caused by free radicals. Vitamins C and E, selenium, carotenoids and polyphenols are among the most antioxidant substances.

BETA-CAROTENE
Carotene precursor of vitamin A. This powerful antioxidant is found mainly in yellow, orange and red fruits and vegetables (for example, carrots, pumpkins and sweet potatoes) as well as in leafy green vegetables (such as spinach and Brussels sprouts), where the pigment is masked by the chlorophyll.

BETAINE
Compound with potentially antidepressive effects.

CALCIUM
Mineral essential to the formation and development of bones and teeth. Not only does calcium strengthen bones, it also plays an important role in healing wounds and muscle contraction and relaxation. It is involved in regulating blood pressure, normalizing the heartbeat and transmitting messages from the nervous system. The best sources of calcium are dairy products and substitutes. Canned fish (such as sardines and salmon) are also good sources if the bones are eaten. Leafy green vegetables, such as broccoli and cabbage, also provide calcium, but in lesser amounts. Calcium from legumes, nuts and seeds is not as easily absorbed by the body as calcium from dairy products.

CARBOHYDRATES
The body's main source of energy. The complex carbohydrates contained, for example, in whole-grain products, vegetables, fruits and legumes are best. A diet with complex carbohydrates can protect against heart disease and stabilize blood sugar.

CAROTENOIDS
Pigments that give fruits and vegetables a yellow, orange or red color. Carotenoids are powerful antioxidants that act preventatively against certain degenerative illnesses. They protect cells exposed to ultraviolet rays from oxidative damage. According to a number of studies, they may slow the growth of cancerous tumors. Carotenoids include lutein and zeaxanthin, lycopene (found in tomatoes), capsanthin (found in red peppers) and beta-carotene, a precursor to vitamin A.

CHOLINE

A B complex vitamin component. Choline promotes proper brain functioning and improves memory; it may slow the progression of Alzheimer's disease and dementia. It is found mainly in egg yolk, but also in liver, meat, fish, peanuts and nuts.

COPPER

A trace element that helps fight against free radicals. Copper also helps in the formation of red blood cells and many hormones. It is found in mollusks and shellfish, meat, nuts, seeds and legumes.

CORTISOL

Hormone secreted by the body in response to chronic stress.

DOPAMINE

Neurotransmitter (sometimes called the pleasure hormone) responsible for keeping the brain alert and active. High dopamine levels seem to promote adventurous behavior, pleasure and thrill seeking and sexual pleasure. Abnormally low levels are associated with a lack of motivation, melancholy and emotional emptiness.

ESSENTIAL FATTY ACIDS

Polyunsaturated fats called essential because the body cannot make them, and they are needed for its functioning and development. *See* Omega-3s.

FIBER

Carbohydrates that the body cannot digest. Fiber arrives intact in the large intestine, where it ferments under the effects of intestinal bacteria. The health benefits of fiber come from this fermentation. It is found in foods of plant origin (foods of animal origin contain virtually no fiber). There are two major families of fiber: soluble fiber and insoluble fiber. *See* Insoluble Fiber *and* Soluble Fiber.

FLAVONOIDS

Phytochemical compounds in the family of polyphenols. Whether isoflavonoids, quercetin, anthocyanins, anthocyanidines, flavonols or flavones, all of these compounds appear to limit oxidative damage caused by free radicals. In addition to reducing inflammation that can lead to atherosclerosis, therefore to heart disease, they can play a role in preventing cancer. Flavonoids are found in colorful fruits and vegetables.

FOLATE

Vitamin B_9, more commonly known as folic acid, is the synthetic form of folate. *See* Vitamin B complex.

FREE RADICALS

Molecules naturally produced by the body through breathing and the digestion of food. While they help the body get rid of certain viruses, germs and bacteria, even its own cells when they are damaged, free radicals become harmful when too many of them are produced. They damage cells and limit their ability to regenerate. This excess of free radicals is called oxidative stress. Our body has an internal antioxidant system that gets rid of free radicals but antioxidants in diet may be of valuable help.

HEME IRON

Type of iron found in animal products. Heme iron (also called haem iron) is the best source of iron for the body, because it is easier to assimilate than plant-based iron.

INSOLUBLE FIBER

Fiber that helps regulate intestinal transit and creates a feeling of fullness. It is found primarily in the peel of fruits and vegetables, whole grains and wheat bran.

IODINE

An essential component of thyroid hormones. They are involved in many functions, including the functioning of the nervous system. The best sources of iodine are shellfish and mollusks (e.g., clams), fish (e.g., cod, haddock) and seaweed, but also pork, chicken, dairy products, eggs, baked goods, salted processed foods and iodized table salt.

IRON

Trace element essential not only to carrying oxygen and the formation of red blood cells, but also to chemical reactions within cells. To better absorb iron, it is a good idea to eat foods rich in vitamin C (e.g., citrus, berries and certain vegetables, such as peppers) in a single meal. There are two types of dietary iron: heme iron and non-heme iron. *See* Heme Iron *and* Non-heme Iron.

LIPIDS

Saturated, polyunsaturated and monounsaturated fatty acids. Lipids provide the body energy and are building blocks for all of the body's cells. They ensure proper brain function and facilitate the absorption of vitamins A, D, E and K. *See* Essential Fatty Acids, Saturated Fatty Acids, Unsaturated Fatty Acids.

LUTEIN AND ZEAXANTHIN

Carotenoid pigments that give vegetables their bright color (yellow, orange, red or green). Abundant in food, lutein and zeaxanthin are essential to good eye health. A diet rich in lutein and zeaxanthin appears to prevent cataracts. The best sources of lutein are leafy green vegetables (e.g., spinach, kale) and eggs. The best sources of zeaxanthin are leafy green vegetables and red pepper.

LYCOPENE

Pigment that gives vegetables a red color. It is the most abundant carotenoid in the human body. Lycopene is a very active antioxidant. It may reduce the risk of prostate cancer and slow its development, and may protect the skin against the free radicals produced by ultraviolet rays. In turn, it also potentially slows skin aging. The best sources are tomatoes and derivatives (e.g., tomato sauce, tomato paste), watermelon, pink or red grapefruit and red pepper.

MAGNESIUM

Mineral that activates over 300 biochemical reactions in the body. Magnesium helps build bones and teeth. It makes muscles and nerves work and maintains a regular heartbeat. Every cell in the body requires magnesium. It is found in green vegetables, legumes, nuts and seeds, cocoa and certain whole-grain products (such as whole wheat bread).

MANGANESE

A trace element that plays an indirect role in a number of metabolic processes and that prevents the damage caused by free radicals. Manganese helps metabolize carbohydrates and fats, in the formation of cartilage and healthy bones and in regulating blood sugar. The best sources are whole grains, nuts and seeds, legumes and certain fruits and vegetables.

METHIONINE

Essential amino acid, i.e., which the body cannot produce and which comes exclusively from diet.

MINERALS

Micronutrients that are indispensable to the proper functioning of the body. These include calcium, magnesium, phosphorus, potassium and sodium.

NEUROTRANSMITTERS

Chemical messengers that ensure the proper functioning of the brain. Without neurotransmitters, we would have no memory or emotions. The two main neurotransmitters for well-being are serotonin and dopamine.

NON-HEME IRON

Type of iron found in plant-based products. The amount of non-heme iron a food delivers depends on the other products consumed in the same meal: for example, meat proteins and vitamin C increase the absorption of non-heme iron from grains, legumes and vegetables. Wine, tea and coffee reduce its absorption.

NUTRIENTS

Substances needed for the body's functioning.

OMEGA-3S

Polyunsaturated fatty acids called essential found in fish and some plants. Fatty fish (e.g., salmon, rainbow trout, mackerel, herring, halibut, tuna, sardines), ground flaxseed and walnuts are good sources of it. It is important to differentiate the three types of omega-3s: alpha-linolenic acid (ALA), mainly from plant sources, eicosapentaenoic acid (EPA) and docosahexaenoic fatty acid (DHA), mainly from marine sources. All of them are beneficial for the body. However, the effects on heart health have been observed particularly with a high intake of omega-3s from fish and fish oil (EPA and DHA). It is a good idea to make it part of your diet two or three times a week. As for omega-3s of plant origin, even though they are not as easy for the body to assimilate, they should be included in your diet.

OXIDATIVE STRESS

An attack that damages the body's cells caused by free radicals. The compounds that fight oxidative stress are called antioxidants. Oxidative stress could be at the source of a number of diseases, including heart disease and cancer.

PHENYLALANINE

Amino acid that helps make dopamine, a neurotransmitter responsible for regulating mood and motivation.

PHOSPHORUS

One of the most important minerals in the body after calcium. Phosphorus is essential to almost all chemical reactions in the cells. It helps maintain bone and tooth health and produces the energy the body needs. Foods high in protein (meat, poultry, fish, dairy products, eggs, legumes, nuts and seeds) and whole grains are the main sources of it. However, the phosphorus contained in food of plant origin (such as grains, legumes and nuts) is less bioavailable than that contained in food of animal origin.

PHYTONUTRIENTS

Substance of plant origin with nutritional value. These are not vitamins or minerals, but pigments or biologically active compounds. Known for their antioxidant properties, phytonutrients may offer protection against premature aging, cardiovascular disease and cancer. They are sulfur compounds, phytosterols, polyphenols (e.g., flavonoids, phenolic acids, tannins), resveratrol and terpenes (e.g., carotenoids, lutein, zeaxanthin, lycopene).

PHYTOSTEROLS

Phytonutrients that lower LDL cholesterol ("bad" cholesterol), preventing heart disease. According to studies, phytosterols may also have anti-cancer properties. They are found in sesame and sunflower seeds, sesame oil and nuts.

POLYPHENOLS

Antioxidants of plant origin. The family of polyphenols, or phenolic compounds, includes a number of phytonutrients such as flavonoids, phenolic acids and tannins.

POTASSIUM

Mineral necessary for muscle contraction, the contraction and dilatation of blood vessels, and the transmission of nerve impulses. It works closely with sodium and is involved in many biochemical reactions in the body. It also contributes to kidney health and, working with sodium, ensures the body's cells are hydrated. The main sources of potassium are fruits and fresh vegetables, but dairy products and legumes also have it.

PROTEIN

Nutrient present in all of the body's cells, including skin, muscles, hair and blood. Protein is indispensable to the functioning of the heart, contributes to tissue growth and repair, participates in the production of antibodies, hormones, neurotransmitters and enzymes involved in many biochemical reactions. Diet must deliver enough protein for the body, which is unable to build up reserves. Food proteins are amino acid chains that are taken apart by the body then rebuilt to form new proteins that perform different functions. During digestion, proteins divide into smaller molecules called amino acids. There are 20 different amino acids and some are considered essential because the body cannot make them. They come exclusively from diet. Complete proteins, i.e., those that contain all the amino acids essential to the proper functioning of the body, are found in products of animal origin (e.g.: meat, fish, eggs and dairy products). Plants (legumes, nuts and seeds) are also good sources of protein, but they are incomplete. Grains also contain incomplete proteins.

QUERCETIN

A particularly antioxidant phytonutrient. Quercetin offers not only protection against cancer but also provides cardiovascular protection. It is also found in onions, berries, dark chocolate and tea.

RESVERATROL

Phytonutrient that is particularly abundant in the skin of red grapes. Resveratrol is a good ally in fighting aging and cancer because it reverses skin damage related to ultraviolet rays. As an antioxidant, it blocks the action of free radicals in the skin. Red grapes and red wine are two primary sources of resveratrol in the diet.

SATURATED FATTY ACIDS

Fatty acids that are normally solid at room temperature. These include foods of animal origin (meat, lard, dairy products), palm and coconut oils and hydrogenated margarine. Some saturated fatty acids are responsible for increased LDL cholesterol ("bad" cholesterol) in the blood.

SELENIUM

Trace element with very high antioxidant capacity. Selenium protects cells against free radicals. It is also involved in the proper functioning of the immune system, allows for the synthesis of testosterone and fosters the production of healthy sperm. Selenium enters the food chain through plants, which draw the mineral from the soil. The amount of selenium in plants depends on where they are grown. Brazil nuts and seafood are good sources of selenium.

SEROTONIN

Neurotransmitter (sometimes called the happiness hormone) that plays an important role in the sense of well-being. Serotonin promotes relaxation, a good mood, serenity, appetite and sleep, while reducing tension, aggression and anger. High serotonin levels promote calm, prudent and considered behavior. Abnormally low levels are associated with irritability, impulsivity and aggression.

SODIUM

Micronutrient that plays a major role in hydrating the body by controlling, along with potassium, water entering and leaving cells. Sodium is essential to the transmission of nerve impulses and enables muscle contraction. While it is indispensable, it should be consumed in moderation. A proper balance is required. Any excess could contribute to an increase in blood pressure, a risk factor for heart disease, and promote the loss of bone mass. Too little sodium can cause undesirable effects (dehydration, nausea, muscle cramps and vertigo). The main sources of sodium are table salt, fish (canned, marinated or smoked), soy sauce, feta cheese, store-bought foods (e.g., canned soup, deli meat), and dehydrated, dried and smoked foods.

SOLUBLE FIBER

Fiber that slows digestion and the assimilation of food. It lowers blood cholesterol and stabilizes blood sugar. It is found in legumes, nuts, fruits and oat bran.

SULFUR COMPOUNDS

Chemical substance often associated with a strong odor. The name of these substances comes from the fact that there are one or more sulfur atoms in their chemical structure. They are found in cabbage, garlic and onion.

TANNINS

Phytonutrients present in certain plants. Tannins protect plants from parasites. These antioxidant substances give food a bitter taste. Tea and red wine are good sources.

THEOBROMINE

Substance with antidepressive effects naturally present in cocoa and chocolate. The term *theobromine* is derived from Theobroma cacao, the generic name for the cacao tree.

TRACE ELEMENTS

Micronutrients present in very small quantities in the body, but indispensable to its proper functioning. They include copper, iron, manganese, molybdenum, selenium and zinc.

TRANS FATTY ACIDS

Polyunsaturated fatty acids naturally present in milk and the meat of ruminants, but that are mostly made artificially through hydrogenation (an industrial process that transforms liquid oil into solid fat). Industrial trans fatty acids raise LDL cholesterol ("bad" cholesterol) in the blood and reduce the level of HDL cholesterol ("good" cholesterol). They are found in shortening, hydrogenated margarine, store-bought cookies and desserts, industrial bakery products, chips, frying oil and frozen french fries.

TRYPTOPHAN

Amino acid transformed into serotonin by the body.

TYROSINE

Amino acid that helps produce dopamine, a neurotransmitter responsible for regulating mood and motivation. A tyrosine deficiency can result in a lack of concentration and motivation.

UNSATURATED FATTY ACIDS

Monounsaturated and polyunsaturated fatty acids that can help reduce blood cholesterol. They are found in oils, nuts and seeds.

VITAMIN A

Vitamin that contributes to good vision, particularly at night. Vitamin A promotes the growth of bones and tissue that cover different parts of the body (cornea, bronchial tubes, intestine, genital mucus and skin) and strengthens the immune system. The main sources of vitamin A are products of animal origin, including butter, whole milk, cheese and eggs.

VITAMIN B COMPLEX

Group of vitamins that include B_1 (thiamine), B_2 (riboflavin), B_3 (niacin), B_5 (pantothenic acid), B_6, B_9 (*see also* Folate) and B_{12}. These vitamins protect nerve cells and contribute to proper brain functioning. In the body, they work together to promote the proper use of nutrients, help liberate energy and reinforce the immune system.

VITAMIN C

Vitamin that is particularly antioxidizing. Vitamin C is known to strengthen the immune system, but it also stimulates the production of collagen, promotes skin elasticity, accelerates scarring, helps repair damaged tissue and enables the absorption of iron in foods. Vitamin C is found mainly in citrus fruit (e.g., orange, lemon and grapefruit), berries and vegetables (e.g., broccoli, kale and red pepper).

VITAMIN D

Vitamin that is essential for fighting osteoporosis. Vitamin D enables the absorption of calcium and attachment to bones. Calcium and vitamin D work together for bone and tooth health. Present in certain foods, it can also be produced by the body through exposure to the ultraviolet rays of the sun. The best dietary sources of vitamin D are fish (e.g., salmon, sardines), cod liver and cod liver oil, egg yolk, cow's milk, enriched yogurt, enriched orange juice, soy milk and enriched almonds.

VITAMIN E

Vitamin with antioxidant properties. Vitamin E protects cells against the effects of free radicals, which are responsible for the damage caused to cells, contributing to the development of heart disease and cancer. Vitamin E is found in almonds, sunflower seeds, nuts, avocado, vegetable oils (e.g., olive, canola and sunflower), wheat germ and certain dark green leafy vegetables (e.g., spinach, Swiss chard).

VITAMIN K

Vitamin that plays an important role in blood clotting. Its name comes from the Danish koagulation. Promoting the formation of bones, vitamin K prevents osteoporosis. It also plays an important role in cognitive function and promotes nerve impulses. The main sources are green vegetables, vegetable oil and soy derivatives (tofu and edamame).

VITAMINS

Essential nutrients found in trace amounts in the body. Vitamins are essential to chemical reactions that shape our physical and mental health.

ZEAXANTHIN

See Lutein and zeaxanthin.

ZINC

Mineral essential to life. Present in almost all cells, zinc is involved in over 100 different enzymatic reactions. It helps the body fight infection, promotes the healing of injuries and wounds and helps maintain taste and smell. It also enables the normal growth of the fetus during pregnancy, as well as growth of children and teens. Zinc is present in many foods: red meat, poultry, legumes, nuts, seafood (particularly oysters), whole grains and dairy products. However, zinc from animal sources is better absorbed than zinc from grains, legumes and vegetables.

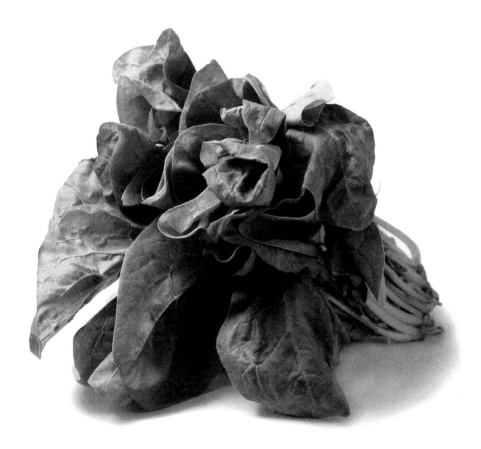

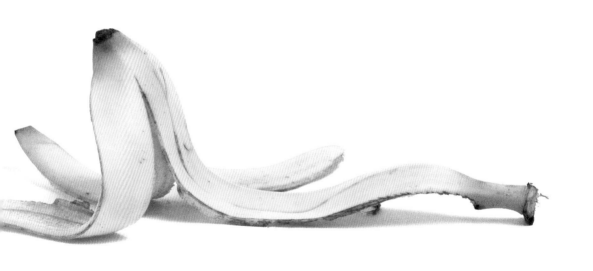

SUPERFOOD
INDEX

ASPARAGUS

AVOCADO

BANANA

BEETS

209

SALMON

SARDINES

SPINACH

SUNFLOWER SEEDS

SWEET POTATO

WALNUTS

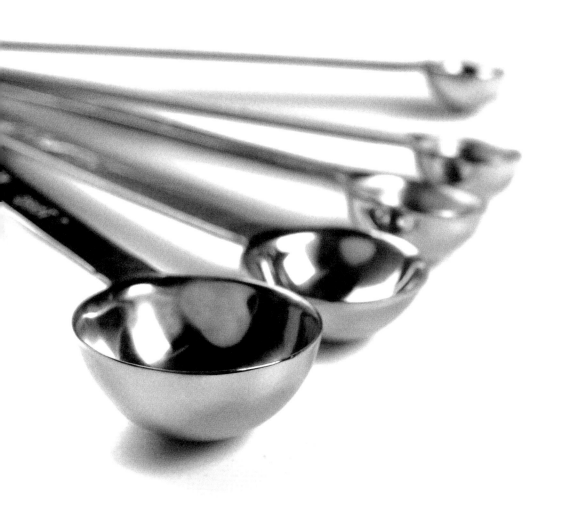

SUPERFOODS ANTI-AGING

Do you want to be healthy for as long as possible and reduce the visible signs of aging? Discover how your diet can make a difference.

This book features 20 anti-aging superfoods and over 50 recipes using these fabulous foods: Grapefruit Elixir, Broccoli Soup, Chicken Salad with Avocado and Walnuts, Maple and Mustard-Crusted Salmon, Seared Scallops and Shrimp with Grapefruit, Chicken with 50 Cloves of Garlic, Lima Bean Wraps, Berries in Red Wine with Spices, Fruity Chocolate Fondue and more.

Superfoods Anti-Aging: everything you need to know to slow down the effects of aging.

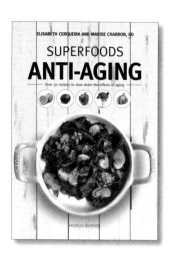

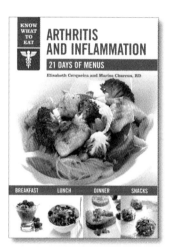

ARTHITIS AND INFLAMMATION

Are your joints swollen and painful? Do you have a hard time getting up in the morning or going up and down stairs? No diet can cure arthritis, but an anti-inflammatory diet can help reduce joint pain.

This guide is specifically designed to help you identifying the best foods for your condition.

Discover delicious recipes that are quick and easy to prepare: Incredible Green Smoothies, Root Vegetable Pâté, Gingery Sweet Potato Soup, Fennel and Orange Salad, Spring Rolls, Kale Stuffed with Poultry and Basmati Rice, Nut-Crusted Salmon, Healthy Truffles, Summer Fruit Salad with Chia Seed and more.

To meet the needs of an even larger audience, the recipes in this book are gluten free.

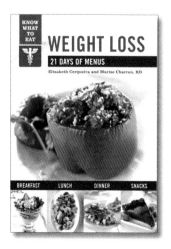

WEIGHT LOSS

Lose weight without drastic dieting, forbidden foods, health risks and, best of all, without regaining the weight you've lost! By changing your lifestyle and adopting healthy eating habits you will be able to manage your weight while enjoying the pleasures of life.

This guide is specifically designed to help you fulfill your nutritional needs without feeling hungry.

Discover recipes that are tasty, simple and quick to prepare: Chicken Quesadillas, Brussels Sprout Chips, Quiche in Quinoa Crust, Marinated Salmon with Mango Salsa, Zucchini Lasagna with Seafood, Portuguese-Style Roast Chicken, Almond-Chocolate Shortcrust Pie, Date Tiramisu and more.